ISBN: 9781081857431

90-DAY
VEGETARIAN DIET
PESCETARIAN
1200-CALORIE

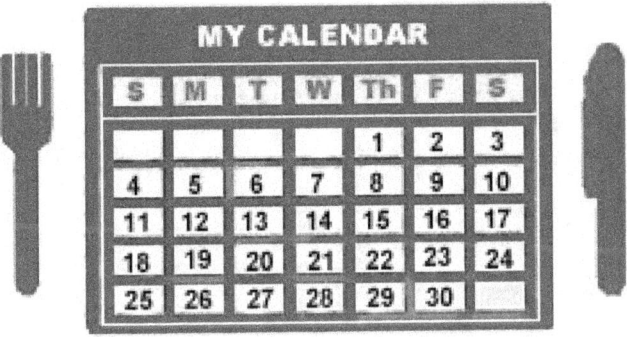

S. Vijay Gupta
Gail Johnson, M.S.

NoPaperPress™

Note: At publication, the off-the-shelf foods used in this book were widely available in most supermarkets. But food products come and go. So if there is a frozen entrée or soup selection in this diet that is out of stock, or that's been discontinued, or perhaps you don't like, or that you forgot to pick up while shopping, please substitute another food that has **approximately** the same caloric value and nutritional content. In this regard, many dieters have found the foods listed in the Appendices at the end of this book to be very helpful.

CONTENTS

1200-Calorie Meal Plans

Recipes & Diet Tips

Day 10b – Lo-Cal Eggplant Parmesan
Day 11 – Mexican Beans and Rice (122)
Day 12 – Fish Dinner Out
Day 13 – Pasta with Marinara Sauce (124)
Day 14a - Smoothie
Day 14b – Frozen Fish Dinner (126)
Day 15 – Spaghetti Squash & Cheese
Day 16 – Baked Red Snapper (128)
Day 17 – Vegetarian Hash
Day 18 – Grilled Swordfish (130)
Day 19 – Pasta-based Dinner Out
Day 20 – Beans & Greens Salad (132)
Day 21 - Frozen Pasta Dinner
Day 22 – Tomato Risotto Salad (134)
Day 23 – Quick Pasta Puttanesca
Day 24 – Four Beans Plus Salad (136)
Day 25 – Tofu with Veggies & Peanuts
Day 26 – Grilled Scallops & Polenta (138)
Day 27 – Fettuccine in Summer Sauce
Day 28 – Frozen Tofu-based Dinner (140)
Day 29 – Healthy Frittata
Day 30 – Portobello Mushroom Burger (142)
Day 31 – Baked Sea Bass
Day 32 – Fish with Orzo (144)
Day 33 – Frozen Vegetarian Dinner
Day 34 – Pasta Rapini   (146)
Day 35 – Vegetarian Dinner Out
Day 36 – Grilled Tilapia (148)
Day 37 – Bulgur & Veggies
Day 38 – Risotto Primavera (150)
Day 39 – Tofu Steak with Veggies
Day 40 – Fish Dinner Out (152)
Day 41 – Pasta e Fagioli
Day 42 – Muffins (154)
Day 43 – Halibut and Corn
Day 44 – Baked Haddock (156)
Day 45 – Quinoa with Veggies Salad
Day 46 – Poached Cod   (158)
Day 47 – Healthy Pasta Salad
Day 48 – Vegetarian Dinner Out (160)

Day 49 – Frozen Pasta-Based Dinner
Day 50 – Pan-Fried Sole (162)
Day 51 – Beans & Greens Salad
Day 52 – Bay Scallops & Snow Peas (164)
Day 53 – Tofu, Bok Choy & Mushroom Stir Fry
Day 54 – Vegetables with Couscous (166)
Day 55 – Hearty Vegetable Soup
Day 56 – Frozen Tofu-based Dinner (168)
Day 57 – Salmon with Mango Salsa
Day 58 – Tofu & Broccoli in Garlic Sauce (170)
Day 59 – Pasta-Based Dinner Out
Day 60 – Cashew Tofu Stir Fry (172)
Day 61 – Shells with Cheese & Walnuts
Day 62 – Curried Eggplant & Tomato (174)
Day 63 – Indian Shahi Paneer
Day 64 – Grilled Scallops & Polenta (176)
Day 65 – Frozen Vegetarian Dinner
Day 66 – Pita Pizza (178)
Day 67 – Fish Dinner Out
Day 68 – Sorba Noodles & Broccoli Rabe (180)
Day 69 – Tofu-Veggie Stir Fry
Day 70 – Baked Cod (182)
Day 71 – Tortellini Pasta & Beans
Day 72 – Pasta-Based Dinner Out (184)
Day 73 – Frozen Fish Dinner
Day 74 – Pasta Pomodoro (186)
Day 75 – Spaghetti Squash
Day 76 – Grilled Scallops (188)
Day 77 – Eggplant Parmesan
Day 78 – Trout with Lemon & Capers (190)
Day 79 – Vegetarian Dinner Out
Day 80 – Vegetable Chili (192)
Day 81 – Frozen Pasta-based Dinner
Day 82 – Avocado & Rice Salad (194)
Day 83 – Hearty Lentil Stew
Day 84 – Black-eyed Peas over Rice (196)
Day 85 – Tina's Healthy Frittata
Day 86 – Tuna & Bean Salad (198)
Day 87 – Pasta Primavera
Day 88 – Frozen Tofu-based Dinner (200)

Appendix A: Vegetarian Background & Nutrition

Appendix B: Vegetarian Soup (208)

Appendix C: Frozen Food Warning

NoPaperPress Paperbacks and eBooks (211)

Disclaimer

The 90-Day Vegetarian Diet blends traditional American cooking with Asian vegetarian concepts. Of course this diet is meatless, but fish, eggs and dairy are allowed. The diet is a Pescetarian version of vegetarianism and features delicious, low calorie, nutritionally balanced vegetarian meals.

A well planned vegetarian diet can provide the same level of nutrients as a meat-eater's diet. In addition, eating meat-free can have real weight-loss benefits because plant-based foods, such as vegetables, beans and whole grains, are loaded with fiber that help you feel satisfied on fewer calories. And many health-care professionals also think that eating a healthy vegetarian diet is one of the best things you can do for your short-term and long-term health.

Vegetarian Types
When deciding what type of vegetarian you want to be, think about what foods you want to include or avoid. There are several vegetarian versions:

1. **Lacto-Ovo Vegetarians** do not eat animal flesh of any kind (including beef, pork, poultry, fish and shellfish) but they do eat eggs and dairy products. This is the most popular vegetarian diet.

2. **Lacto-Vegetarians** do not eat animal flesh of any kind (including beef, pork, poultry, fish and shellfish) and do not eat meat or eggs – but do consume dairy products.

3. **Ovo-Vegetarians** do not eat animal flesh of any kind (including beef, pork, poultry, fish and shellfish) and do not eat meat or dairy products – but do eat eggs.

4. **Pesceterians** do not eat meat or poultry but do eat eggs, dairy and fish. Some Pesceterians also eat other seafood (shrimp, scallops, etc.). People often adopt this diet for health reasons, or as a stepping stone to a fully vegetarian diet. This vegetarian version is sometimes called Semi-Vegetarian.

5. **Vegans** are strict vegetarians who do not eat meat of any kind and also do not eat eggs, dairy products, or processed foods containing these or other animal-derived ingredients. Many vegans also refrain from eating foods that are made using animal products even though the food may not contain animal products in the finished product, such as sugar and some wines.

With this book, NoPaperPress publishes a popular vegetarian variant: the **Pesceterian Vegetarian Diet** that includes fish, eggs and dairy products. And all NoPaperPress vegetarian diet books come in 90-day, 30-day and 7-day editions. For background and nutritional information and more on vegetarianism see **Appendix A** (page 203).

Why You Lose Weight

Most experts agree that when the energy value of the food you eat minus waste, equals the sum of your basal metabolic energy plus the energy you expend during physical activity, you will neither gain nor lose weight. They also agree that when you have an energy imbalance, you will either gain or lose weight. In general then:

- **Weight Maintenance** occurs when your food energy intake equals the total energy you expend in daily living. In this case your weight remains stable, i.e., you neither gain nor lose weight.

- **Weight Gain** occurs when your food energy intake is greater than the total energy you expend in daily living. In this case your body stores the extra energy as fat.

- **Weight Loss** occurs when your food energy intake is less than the total energy you expend in daily living. In this case your body converts stored fat (and in some cases muscle) into energy.

The measure of energy, whether in the form of food, physical activity, or heat, is the kilocalorie (hereafter simply called the Calorie). As already mentioned, weight loss occurs when you eat fewer calories than the calories you use in your day-to-day living. This difference in calories is referred to as your calorie deficit. How much weight you lose depends on the magnitude of your calorie deficit. (In technical terms, **the calorie deficit, or calorie difference, is the driving force for weight change**.)

Most people on a weight-loss diet want to know how much weight they will lose – and how fast. Simple metabolic calculations make a rough estimate possible. Physiologists have long known that to lose one pound requires a deficit of approximately 3,500 Calories. Therefore, if a person's total calorie deficit over time is known, their weight loss over time can be calculated. (See "**Expected Weight Loss**" on page 10.) **In summary, if you eat and exercise such that you have a calorie deficit you will lose weight!**

The Best Weight Loss Diets

According to the late Dr. Jean Mayer, of Tufts University's Department of Nutrition, a really good weight-loss diet must have the following three characteristics:

1) The diet must provide you with an understanding of weight control as well as the knowledge you need to reduce your weight to the desired level.
2) The diet must help you remain healthy while you are losing weight.
3) The diet must lead you to a healthier way of eating and exercising that will, in the long term, help you keep off the weight you have lost.

Why a 90-Day Diet?

Experts agree that a diet that promotes weight loss over a relatively longer time period is healthier and the weight loss is likely to be more permanent. These experts recommend you choose a nutritious diet that results in a weight loss of approximately 2 pounds per week – which amounts to about 26 lbs in 90 days. The *90-Day Vegetarian (Pescetarian) Diet* fits the bill!

Expected Weight Loss

On the *90-Day Vegetarian Diet (Pescetarian) – 1200 Calorie Edition*, **most women lose 23 to 33 pounds.** Smaller women, older women and less active women lose a bit less and larger women, younger women and more active women often lose much more.

On the *90-Day Vegetarian Diet (Pescetarian) – 1200 Calorie Edition*, **most men lose 35 to 45 pounds**. Smaller men, older men and less active men will lose a tad less and larger men, younger men and more active men frequently lose much more.

Exactly how much weight you will lose depends on how much you weigh, your age and your activity level. For the full story see *Weight Control - U.S. Edition* by Vincent W. Antonetti, Ph.D., a book also published by NoPaperPress.

90-Day Diet Info

The *90-Day Vegetarian Diet* contains meal plans, recipes and guidance for 90 fat-melting days! How long you stay on the diet, 10 days, 45 days, or all 90 days – depends on how much weight you want to lose.

Day 1 of the diet starts on page 19. Associated with each of the 90 days is a "**Recipe of the Day**" (page 110) and a "Diet Tip of the Day."

Even though the *90-Day Vegetarian Diet* adheres to the United States Department of Agriculture balanced diet recommendations, this diet may not be appropriate for everyone, such as individuals with illnesses like heart disease, diabetes, food allergies, etc. Make sure you check with your physician before starting this diet, or any diet.

First a Medical Exam

Everyone should at the very least have a medical assessment, or exam, before starting a weight loss diet. Why? You need to make sure your health will allow you to lower your caloric intake and increase your physical activity. Depending on your age and state of health, the medical checkup may be as simple as a visit to a physician who is familiar with your medical history, or it may be a thorough physical exam.

The physician conducting the medical exam should be made aware of and should approve the specific weight loss diet you're planning. Additionally, if you are going to engage in some sort of physical activity in conjunction with this diet and especially if you have been totally inactive, or if you have or suspect you have cardiovascular disease or other health problems, or if you are obese, or if you are 40 or older, before embarking on the physical fitness portion of your weight control program you should have a stress test supervised by a physician. Finally, your physician can tell you how much and what type of exercise is right for you, how much you should weigh, and prescribe a realistic weight- loss goal.

Eat Smart

No single food can supply all the nutrients you need in the amounts you need. The most important factors in nutrition are variety, variety, variety! **Variety is the key to a nutritious diet.** As a means of setting strategies for food selection, the U.S. Department of Health and Human Services and the Department of Agriculture issue Dietary Guidelines every five years. The latest Dietary Guidelines describe a healthy diet as one that:
- Emphasizes fruits, vegetables, whole grains, and fat-free or low-fat milk products.
- Includes fish, beans and nuts.
- Is low in saturated fats, trans fats, cholesterol, salt (sodium) and added sugars.

The latest guidelines encourage adults to consume a variety of nutrient-dense foods and beverages within their caloric needs. The afore mentioned U.S. government agencies recommend how much should be eaten from each of the basic food groups to meet your caloric goal – whether you are trying to lose weight or maintain weight.

Even though most adults can get all the vitamins and minerals they need by merely consuming a variety of nutritious foods, many physicians recommend a daily multi-vitamin/mineral supplement – just in case you don't eat the way you should. Be aware that some micronutrients, such as the fat-soluble vitamin A, can be harmful if taken in large quantities. To be safe your multi-vitamin/mineral supplement should contain no more than 100 percent of the recommended dietary allowance (RDA) for each vitamin or mineral. Generally, you don't need the high doses in multi-vitamin/mineral supplements labeled "therapeutic" or "extra-strength." There may be medical reasons for taking larger amounts of a vitamin or mineral than the RDA provides, but check with your doctor first.

Tossed Salad

One of the dinner mainstays in the *90-Day Vegetarian Diet* is a "Tossed Salad." To prepare your "Tossed Salad" start with a bowl that has a volume of <u>at least</u> 16 ounces, or 2 cups. First add about 1 cup of either green leaf lettuce, Romaine lettuce or a Mesclun mix. Then add at least a half cup of other veggies such as broccoli, celery, cucumber, spinach, or watercress. This vegetable combination will, on average, total about 35 Calories.

You'll be eating a "Tossed Salad" just about every day at dinnertime. Remember that variety is the key to a nutritious diet. So be sure to vary the ingredients of the salad.

Top your "Tossed Salad" with <u>1½ tablespoons of any light salad dressing</u> available at your local supermarket that contains no more than 25 Calories per tablespoon. Some of our favorite light salad dressings are:
- **Kraft Light Done Right House Italian**
- **Newman's Lighten Up! Balsamic Vinaigrette**
- **Wishbone Just 2 Good Honey Dijon**

Your "Tossed Salad" with salad dressing will cost you roughly 70 Calories but will be packed with lots of health-giving vitamins, minerals and fiber. (Remember to check the labels of all processed products to assure that they are vegetarian.)

About Bread

First understand that bread, more specifically whole-grain breads, are good sources of complex carbohydrates and dietary fiber, as well as the B vitamins (thiamin, riboflavin, niacin, and folate), vitamin E, and minerals (iron, magnesium and selenium). In recent years, however, sliced bread loaves have gotten larger, as have the bread slices inside these loaves. Just a few years ago the standard slice of bread contained about 65 to 70 Calories – now most are 100 plus Calories.

The 90-*Day Vegetarian Diet* requires whole-grain bread at 70 Calories per slice. Quite a few bakers sell thin sliced or "light" sliced bread. The difficult part is finding a whole grain thin sliced or "light" bread (with about 70 Calories per slice). Whatever the brand, make sure the first word in the Ingredients list is "whole." "Pepperidge Farm Small Slice 100% Whole Wheat" is a good choice. It's whole grain, has 70 Calories per slice and it tastes good too.

Substituting Foods

If there is a food listed in the *90-Day Vegetarian Diet* that you don't like, or perhaps that you forgot to pick up while shopping, you probably can exchange or substitute another food in its place – a technique used by dieticians. Exchanging a food listed in a diet for another food with approximately equal caloric value and nutritional content is the foundation of many successful long-term diets. Substitution possibilities are almost endless but have to be done carefully. The easiest substitutions are those within the same food group, such as exchanging one vegetable variety for another, or a glass of milk for a cup of yogurt. More sophisticated exchanges cross food groups, such as replacing 3½ ounces of tofu with a tablespoon of peanut butter on a piece of whole-wheat bread. Both foods are complete protein and both contain about 175 Calories. (Refer to a good calorie table online.) With some understanding and experience, you can use this table to help you substitute foods called for in the *90-Day Vegetarian Diet* with equal calorie foods from the same food group.

 Breakfast: You may substitute any cereal for any other wholesome cereal. For example, if you're not crazy about having Shredded Wheat for breakfast on Day 6, substitute Wheat Chex or Cheerios, etc. But remember to adjust the amount of cereal to account for the calorie difference between brands. If you don't like the soft-boiled egg called for on Day 9, cook a fried egg instead. And if Cantaloupe is on the menu but is not in season, replace cantaloupe with a half cup of orange juice – both contain about 50 Calories.

 Snacks: Again, where 6 ounces of yogurt is specified you may substitute an 8-ounce glass of skim milk, but to maintain a nutritionally balanced diet keep this snack a dairy selection. Similarly, when fruit is on the agenda, you may select any type of fruit but do not stray from the fruit group. Nuts and popcorn can be interchanged at will. Specified convenient brand-name snacks, such as Skinny Cow ice cream, Kashi Granola bars, Nabisco 100 Calorie Pack cookies and Orville Redenbacher's Smart Pop Popcorn should be widely available but other equivalent brands may be substituted if need be. Just make sure the substitute snack has the same calorie count, or very close, to the specified snack.

Two Nights – No Cooking

Everyone deserves a break from the grind of preparing dinner after coming home from work. So the *90-Day Vegetarian Diet* gives you two days off per week! Notice that one night a week the meal plan calls for a frozen dinner and on a second night during the week you're encouraged to eat out. There are, however, some rules and caveats involved – these are covered in the next two sections.

Frozen Dinner Rules

In general, a frozen dinner should not be a meal in itself. Make sure you add a salad, fruit, bread etc. The frozen dinner you choose should come with at least one cup of cooked vegetables. If your frozen dinner doesn't measure up, add your own frozen, fresh or canned vegetables. And look for dinners with no more than 800 mg of sodium. In addition, make sure the dinner you choose has no more than 30 percent of the daily value for total fat. Some reasonably good frozen dinner choices are:
  – Amy's: Asian Noodle Stir-Fry (300 Calories)
  – Amy's: Indian Vegetable Korma (310 Calories)
  – Amy's: Tofu Scramble (320 Calories)
  – Lean Cuisine: Shrimp Alfredo (200 Calories)
  – Smart Ones: Pasta Primavera (250 Calories)
  And on the days when a frozen dinner is specified, you will also be given a calorie goal for the frozen dinner. For example, Day 5 calls for frozen fish dinner with a maximum allowable 340 Calories. If you choose a frozen fish dinner that contains less than 340 Calories, you may spend the unused calories any way you wish.

  Moreover, on those nights when you just don't have the energy or time to cook, you can always substitute a frozen dinner for the "Recipe of the Day" or the entree listed in the meal plan. For example, Day 2 calls for Herb-Crusted Cod for dinner. The total calorie count for dinner is 520. In place of the cod, any combination of a frozen fish dinner and side dishes (salads, etc) with a total calorie content close to 520 would be an acceptable, albeit not as tasty, alternative.

Eating Out Challenges

On this diet, you are encouraged to eat out once a week. When you're on a diet, however, eating in a restaurant can be a challenge, even in a vegetarian establishment, because most restaurant portions are huge, and can easily total more than 1,000 Calories. On the *90-Day Vegetarian Diet*, a dinner type (i.e., fish, tofu, pasta, etc) and a calorie target are specified.

For example Day 7 of the 1,200 Calorie diet calls for dinner in a vegetarian restaurant and allows you 530 Calories.

First, you need to choose a restaurant where you have a fighting chance to achieve your calorie goal. Next, order something simple, such as stir-fried tofu with steamed vegetables and brown rice. Tell the waiter you want no sauce, no gravy, nothing added. Then, knowing your calorie objective, and that most stir-fried tofu have less than 35 Calories per ounce, most steamed vegetable servings average approximately 50 Calories per cup, and rice is about 100 Calories per ½ cup, decide how much to eat – and take the remainder home. If fresh fruit is not an option, pass on dessert and have the evening snack specified in the *90-Day Vegetarian Diet* meal plan for that day.

On the days a fish dinner is specified, order broiled fish, and note that most broiled fish are about 50 Calories per ounce. On days when pasta is specified, always order pasta with a marinara sauce or pasta primavera. Generally pasta is 45 Calories per ounce and marinara sauce about 70 Calories per ½ cup.

When you eat out, we recommend you use a calculator app on your smart phone to add up the calories in your meal. And keep a file on your phone with the approximate Calories per ounce of the food you are likely to eat when dinning at a restaurant.

90-Day Diet Notes

1) If desired, skim milk and a sugar substitute may be added to coffee or tea. And soy or almond milk may be used instead of cow's milk.

2) Fried eggs or scrambled eggs should be cooked in a pan coated with a non-stick cooking spray. Hard-boiled eggs may be substituted for fried, scrambled or soft-boiled eggs.

3) Cereals should be whole grain and unsweetened. At the top of the list are Old-fashioned Oatmeal, Wheatena and Shredded Wheat. Among other reasonably healthy choices are Cheerios, Wheat Chex, Wheaties, some Kashi cereals and Farina. When blueberries are in season, you may add **blueberries instead of raisins** to your cereal. (Substitution ratio = 2 blueberries for one raisin.)

4) Bread may be either plain or toasted whole grain, such as whole wheat, whole rye or pumpernickel. Look for whole grain varieties that contain 70 Calories per slice. If desired, bread may be sprayed with a zero-calorie butter substitute. BUT NO BUTTER!

5) When canned or microwaveable soup is specified, have only one serving (8 ounces) unless otherwise noted. (Cans and microwaveable bowls usually contain about two servings.)

6) Use freely as desired: clear unsweetened coffee, clear unsweetened tea, water, seltzer water and any diet soda, clear soups without fat, bouillon, and seasonings such as mustard, cinnamon, dill, herbs, red and black pepper, curry, vinegar, lemon juice and sections, and dill and sour pickles.

7) When canned tuna or salmon is specified, use only fish packed in water.

8) An unlimited amount of green salad may be eaten, but the salad dressing should be as specified.

9) In place of skim milk, you may substitute almond or light soy milk.

10) If it's more convenient, any food item may be moved to any part of the day and combined with any meal or snack.

11) If you cannot find the exact item called for in the diet (because it's out of stock or discontinued), substitute a comparable food (of the same type and close caloric value).

12) Although it's recommended that you follow the diet days as specified, it's fine to occasionally skip a day and/or pick and choose the days you prefer. (Nutritionally, each day stands on its own.)

13) NoPaperPress works hard to keep the information in this book up to date. But we recommend that you check the labels of all processed products in this diet to assure that they are still truly vegetarian.

14) After you complete the 90th day on the diet, if you still want to lose more weight you may repeat the diet by starting over at Day 1.

Keeping It Off

Within five years, more than 90 percent of all dieters regain every pound they have lost. Why? In most cases it's because after losing weight most people eventually revert to their pre-diet eating and exercising habits, and this inevitably leads to their regaining the weight they lost – and often more. Obviously after a diet you weigh less. The fact is the less you weigh, the less you need to eat to sustain your lower weight.

A study, published in the *Annals of Internal Medicine*, that followed 4,000 people for three decades suggests that in the long term, 90 percent of men and 70 percent of women will become overweight. Interestingly, half of the men and women in the study, who had made it well into adulthood without a weight problem, ultimately also became overweight and a third actually became obese. The point being that you can never become complacent. You must continually watch your weight because we are all at risk of becoming overweight.

The key to long-term weight control success is knowledge and understanding, combined of course with desire and self-discipline. Once you reach your weight goal, I suggest you read ***Weight Maintenance - U.S. Edition*** by Vincent Antonetti, Ph.D. (also published by NoPaperPress) – absolutely the best weight maintenance book on the market.

1200 Calorie Meal Plans

Day 1 1200 Calorie Meal Plan

BREAKFAST	Calories	Totals
Orange juice (½ cup)	50	
Scrambled egg (See Notes - page 15)	80	
Whole-grain toast (1 slice) (page 12)	70	
Coffee (See Notes)	10	210 Cal
SNACK		
Coffee or tea	10	10 Cal
LUNCH		
Peanut butter (1 Tbsp) on 1 slice GF bread	170	
Skim milk (4 oz)	45	
Water	0	215 Cal
SNACK		
Fresh fruit in season (apple, peach, etc)	70	70 Cal
DINNER		
Crumbly-Tofu Scramble (Day 1 Recipe - page 19)	240	
Five small white potatoes - roasted	250	
Large tossed salad + 1½ Tbsp low-cal dressing (page	70	
Water	0	560 Cal
SNACK		
Graham crackers (4 squares)	120	
Coffee or tea	10	130 Cal
		1195 Cal

Day 2   1200 Calorie Meal Plan

BREAKFAST	Calories	Totals
Orange juice (½ cup)	50	
Wheaties (¾ cup) + ½ cup skim milk + ½ banana	190	
Whole-grain toast (1 slice)	70	
Coffee	10	320 Cal
SNACK		
Fresh fruit in season (apple, pear, etc)	70	
Coffee or tea	10	80 Cal
LUNCH		
Soup (Appendix B - page 208)	60	
Sliced hard-boiled egg on 1 slice bread	150	
Pickle spear	0	
Lettuce & tomato slices	20	
Hot or iced tea	10	240 Cal
SNACK		
Coffee or tea	10	10 Cal
DINNER		
Baked Herb-Crusted Cod (Day 2 Recipe - page 20)	230	
Spinach (½ cup) steamed with garlic & drizzled	100	
Asparagus (8 spear cooked & drained)	25	
Baked potato (medium size) (No Butter!)	100	
Whole-grain bread (1 slice)	70	
Water with lemon wedge	10	535 Cal
SNACK		
Coffee or tea	10	10 Cal
		1195 Cal

Day 3 1200 Calorie Meal Plan

BREAKFAST	Calories	Totals
Fresh or frozen strawberries (½ cup)	25	
French toasted English Muffin (Day 3a Recipe page112)	270	
Light syrup (1 Tbsp)	30	
Coffee	10	335 Cal
SNACK		
Coffee or tea	10	10 Cal
LUNCH		
Salad (3 oz canned tuna, 1 tsp Evoo, onions, celery)	175	
Lettuce & tomato wedges	20	
Rye bread (1 slice)	70	
Fresh fruit in season (apple, peach, etc)	70	
Coffee or tea	10	345 Cal
SNACK		
Coffee or tea	10	10 Cal
DINNER		
Polenta-stuffed peppers (Day 3b Recipe - page 113)	290	
Large tossed salad + 1½ Tbsp low-cal dressing (page	70	
Water	0	370 Cal
SNACK		
Skinny Cow Ice Cream Sandwich	140	
Coffee or tea	10	150 Cal
		1210 Cal

Day 4   1200 Calorie Meal Plan

BREAKFAST	Calories	Totals
Grapefruit (½)	75	
Cheerios (1 cup) + ½ cup skim milk	160	
Coffee	10	245 Cal
SNACK		
Fresh fruit in season (peach, plum, etc)	70	
Coffee or tea	10	80 Cal
LUNCH		
Cottage cheese (1 cup low fat)	180	
Large tossed salad with 1½ Tbsp low-cal dressing	70	
Water	0	250 Cal
SNACK		
Handful unsalted mixed nuts	100	100 Cal
DINNER		
Easy Penne (Day 4 Recipe - page 114)	375	
Italian or French bread (1 slice)	80	
Water	0	455 Cal
SNACK		
Graham crackers (2 squares)	60	
Coffee or tea	10	70 Cal
		1200 Cal

22

Day 5 1200 Calorie Meal Plan

BREAKFAST	Calories	Totals
Cantaloupe (½ medium)	50	
Fried egg	80	
Toasted raisin bread (1 slice)	75	
Coffee	10	215 Cal
SNACK		
Coffee or tea	10	10 Cal
LUNCH		
Soup (Appendix B - page 208)	140	
Small whole-grain roll	80	
Lettuce and sliced tomato + 1 Tbsp low-cal dressing	45	
Canned pineapple (½ cup, no-sugar-added juice)	40	
Hot or iced tea	10	315 Cal
SNACK		
Yogurt (6 oz nonfat, any flavor)	90	
Coffee or tea	10	100 Cal
DINNER		
Frozen Vegetarian dinner (Day 5 Recipe - page 115)	340	
Large tossed salad with 1½ Tbsp low-cal dressing	70	
Whole-grain bread (1 slice)	70	
Fresh fruit in season (apple, peach, etc)	70	
Water	0	550 Cal
SNACK		
Coffee or tea	10	10 Cal
		1200 Cal

Day 6 1200 Calorie Meal Plan

BREAKFAST	Calories	Totals
Tomato juice (½ cup)	20	
Shredded Wheat (1 cup) + ½ cup skim milk + ½ banana	265	
Coffee	10	295 Cal
SNACK		
Coffee or tea	10	10 Cal
LUNCH		
Salad – 3 oz canned salmon, 1 tsp Evoo, onions & celery	200	
Small whole-grain roll	80	
Lettuce	0	
Hot or iced tea	10	290 Cal
SNACK		
Coffee or tea	10	10 Cal
DINNER		
Pizza (Day 6 Recipe - page 116)	350	
Large tossed salad with 1½ Tbsp low-cal dressing	70	
Fresh fruit in season (apple, plum, etc)	70	
Water	0	490 Cal
SNACK		
100-Calorie Pack Cookies*	100	
Coffee or tea	10	110 Cal
* Such as Nabisco Oreo/Chips Ahoy/etc		1205 Cal

Day 7 1200 Calorie Meal Plan

BREAKFAST	Calories	Totals
Cantaloupe (½ medium)	50	
Oatmeal (½ cup dry) + ½ cup skim milk + 15 raisins*	220	
Coffee	10	280 Cal
SNACK		
Coffee or tea	10	10 Cal
LUNCH		
Soup (Appendix B - page 208)	90	
Grilled cheese sandwich (2 slices 2% cheese)	240	
Lettuce and sliced tomato	20	
Pickle spear	0	
Hot or iced tea	10	360 Cal
SNACK		
Coffee or tea	10	10 Cal
DINNER		
Eat Out – Vegetarian restaurant (Day 7 Recipe -page 117)		
Max allowable calories	530	530 Cal
SNACK		
Coffee or tea	10	10 Cal
* See page 15 re substituting blueberries for raisins.		1200 Cal

Day 8 1200 Calorie Meal Plan

BREAKFAST	Calories	Totals
Cantaloupe (½ medium)	50	
Wheaties (¾ cup) + ½ cup skim milk + ½ banana	190	
Coffee	10	250 Cal
SNACK		
Fresh fruit in season (peach, plum, etc)	70	
Coffee or tea	10	80 Cal
LUNCH		
Subway 6" (Veggie Delite)*	190	
Banana (medium)	100	
Hot or iced tea	10	300 Cal
* Half whole-grain roll		
SNACK		
Coffee or tea	10	10 Cal
DINNER		
Baked salmon with salsa (Day 8 Recipe - page 118)	215	
Baked summer squash and zucchini	40	
Medium tomato - sliced	20	
Brown rice (½ cup – after cooking)	100	
Large tossed salad with 1½ Tbsp low-cal dressing	70	
Water with lemon wedge	10	455 Cal
SNACK		
Graham crackers (2 squares)	60	
Skim milk (4 oz)	45	105 Cal
		1200 Cal

Day 9   1200 Calorie Meal Plan

BREAKFAST	Calories	Totals
Orange juice (½ cup)	50	
Soft-boiled egg	80	
Whole grain toast (1 slice)	70	
Coffee	10	210 Cal
SNACK		
Yogurt (6 oz nonfat, any flavor)	90	
Coffee or tea	10	100 Cal
LUNCH		
Salad (3 oz canned tuna, 1 tsp Evoo, onions, celery)	175	
Lettuce & tomato wedges + rye bread (1 slice)	90	
Coffee or tea	10	275 Cal
SNACK		
Handful unsalted mixed nuts	100	100 Cal
DINNER		
Veggie burger – (1 patty) (Day 9 Recipe - page 119)	100	
Low-fat cheddar cheese (1 thin slice)	50	
Seeded hamburger roll	140	
Beets (3 small, boiled, skinned & sliced)	45	
Fresh fruit in season (apple, peach, etc)	70	
Water	0	405 Cal
SNACK		
100-Calorie Pack Cookies	100	
Coffee or tea	10	110 Cal
		1200 Cal

Day 10 1200 Calorie Meal Plan

BREAKFAST	Calories	Totals
Orange juice (½ cup)	50	
Wild blueberry pancakes (Day 10a Recipe - page 120)	190	
Light syrup (1½ Tbsp)	45	
Coffee	10	295 Cal
SNACK		
Coffee or tea	10	10 Cal
LUNCH		
Peanut butter (2 Tbsp) 2 slices bread	340	
Skim milk (4 oz)	45	
Fresh fruit in season (apple, plum, etc)	70	455 Cal
SNACK		
Coffee or tea	10	10 Cal
DINNER		
Lo-Cal Eggplant Parmesan (Day 10b Recipe page 121)	270	
Large tossed salad with 1½ Tbsp low-cal dressing	70	
Italian or French bread (1 slice)	80	
Water	0	430 Cal
SNACK		
Coffee or tea	10	10 Cal
		1200 Cal

Day 11 1200 Calorie Meal Plan

BREAKFAST	Calories	Totals
Fresh sliced orange	75	
Cheerios (1 cup) + ½ cup skim milk + about 15 raisins	190	
Coffee	10	275 Cal
SNACK		
Coffee or tea	10	10 Cal
LUNCH		
Cottage cheese (1 cup low fat)	180	
Large tossed salad with 1½ Tbsp low-cal dressing	70	
Small whole-grain roll	80	
Hot or iced tea	10	340 Cal
SNACK		
Handful unsalted mixed nuts	100	100 Cal
DINNER		
Mexican Beans and Rice (Day 11 Recipe - page 122)	270	
Green beans (¼ lb – steamed)	25	
Whole-grain bread (1 slice)	70	
Water	0	365 Cal
SNACK		
100-Calorie Pack Cookies	100	
Coffee or tea	10	110 Cal
		1200 Cal

Day 12   1200 Calorie Meal Plan

BREAKFAST	Calories	Totals
Orange juice (½ cup)	50	
Scrambled egg	80	
Whole-grain toast (1 slice)	70	
Coffee	10	210 Cal
SNACK		
Yogurt (6 oz nonfat, any flavor)	90	
Coffee or tea	10	100 Cal
LUNCH		
Soup (Appendix B - page 208)	140	
Tomato slices + ¼ cup chopped fresh basil & 1 tsp Evoo	60	
Whole-grain bread (1 slice)	70	
Hot or iced tea	10	280 Cal
SNACK		
Coffee or tea	10	10 Cal
DINNER		
Eat Out – Fish dinner (Day 12 Recipe - page 123)		
Max allowable calories	595	595 Cal
SNACK		
Coffee or tea	10	10 Cal
		1205 Cal

Day 13   1200 Calorie Meal Plan

BREAKFAST	Calories	Totals
Orange juice (½ cup)	50	
Shredded Wheat (1 cup) + ½ cup skim milk + ½ banana	260	
Coffee	10	320 Cal
SNACK		
Handful unsalted mixed nuts	100	100 Cal
LUNCH		
Egg salad (1 hard-boiled egg + 1 Tbsp light mayo)	125	
Small whole-grain roll	80	
Lettuce and sliced tomato with 1 Tbsp low-cal	45	
Hot or iced tea	10	260 Cal
SNACK		
Coffee or tea	10	10 Cal
DINNER		
Pasta - Marinara sauce (Day 13 Recipe - page 124)	225	
Large tossed salad with 1½ Tbsp low-cal dressing	70	
Fresh fruit in season (peach, plum, etc)	70	
Italian or French bread (1 slice)	80	
Water	0	445 Cal
SNACK		
Graham crackers (2 squares)	60	
Coffee or tea	10	70 Cal
		1205 Cal

Day 14 1200 Calorie Meal Plan

BREAKFAST	Calories	Totals
Cantaloupe (½ medium)	50	
Low-Cal Smoothie (Day 14a Recipe - page 125)	220	
Coffee	10	280 Cal
SNACK		
Fresh fruit in season (apple, peach, etc)	70	
Coffee or tea	10	80 Cal
LUNCH		
Grilled Swiss cheese sandwich (2 oz low-fat cheese)	320	
Pickle spear	0	
Hot or iced tea	10	330 Cal
SNACK		
Coffee or tea	10	10 Cal
DINNER		
Frozen Fish dinner (Day 14b Recipe - page 126)	300	
Large tossed salad with 1½ Tbsp low-cal dressing	70	
Water with lemon wedge	10	380 Cal
SNACK		
Popcorn Mini Bag*	110	
Coffee or tea	10	120 Cal
* Such as Orville Redenbacher's Smart Pop		1200 Cal

Day 15 1200 Calorie Meal Plan

BREAKFAST	Calories	Totals
Fresh or frozen strawberries (1 cup)	50	
French toasted English Muffin Day 3a Recipe - page112	270	
Light syrup (1 Tbsp)	30	
Coffee	10	360 Cal
SNACK		
Yogurt (6 oz nonfat, any flavor)	90	
Coffee or tea	10	100 Cal
LUNCH		
Salad (3 oz canned tuna, 1 tsp Evoo, onions, celery)	175	
Rye bread (1 slice)	70	
Coffee or tea	10	255 Cal
SNACK		
Coffee or tea	10	10 Cal
DINNER		
Spaghetti squash & cheese (Day 15 Recipe - page 127)	300	
Brown rice (½ cup – after cooking)	100	
Steamed broccoli (1 cup – after cooking)	50	
Water with lemon wedge	10	460 Cal
SNACK		
Coffee or tea	10	10 Cal
		1195 Cal

Day 16   1200 Calorie Meal Plan

BREAKFAST	Calories	Totals
Orange juice (½ cup)	50	
Kashi GoLean (1 cup) + ½ cup skim milk + ½ banana	235	
Coffee	10	295 Cal
SNACK		
Fresh fruit in season (apple, plum, etc)	70	
Coffee or tea	10	80 Cal
LUNCH		
Soup (Appendix B - page 208)	100	
Small whole-grain roll	80	
Lettuce and sliced tomato with 1 Tbsp low-cal	45	
Hot or iced tea	10	235 Cal
SNACK		
Coffee or tea	10	10 Cal
DINNER		
Baked red snapper (Day 16 Recipe - page 128)	215	
Wild rice mix (Day 16 Recipe)	160	
Green beans & tomato	75	
Water	0	450 Cal
SNACK		
Popcorn Mini Bag	110	
Coffee or tea	10	120 Cal
		1190 Cal

Day 17   1200 Calorie Meal Plan

BREAKFAST	Calories	Totals
Cantaloupe (½ medium)	50	
Fried egg	80	
Toasted raisin bread (1 slice)	75	
Coffee	10	215 Cal
SNACK		
Yogurt (6 oz nonfat, any flavor)	90	
Coffee or tea	10	100 Cal
LUNCH		
Soup (Appendix B - page 208)	160	
Lettuce & tomato sandwich (Tbsp light mayo)	170	
Cucumber slices and carrots and celery sticks	15	
Hot or iced tea	10	355 Cal
SNACK		
Handful unsalted mixed nuts	100	
Coffee or tea	10	110 Cal
DINNER		
Vegetarian hash (Day 17 Recipe - page 129)	320	
Whole-grain bread (1 slice)	70	
Water with lemon wedge	10	400 Cal
SNACK		
Coffee or tea	10	10 Cal
		1190 Cal

Day 18   1200 Calorie Meal Plan

BREAKFAST	Calories	Totals
Grapefruit (½)	75	
Cheerios (1 cup) + ½ cup skim milk + about 15 raisins	190	
Coffee	10	275 Cal
SNACK		
Coffee or tea	10	10 Cal
LUNCH		
Cottage cheese (1 cup low fat)	180	
Large tossed salad with 1½ Tbsp low-cal dressing	70	
Small whole-grain roll	80	
Hot or iced tea	10	340 Cal
SNACK		
Handful unsalted mixed nuts	100	
Coffee or tea	10	110 Cal
DINNER		
Grilled swordfish (Day 18 Recipe - page 130)	250	
Grilled potatoes (Day 18 Recipe)	100	
Grilled cherry tomatoes (Day 18 Recipe)	45	
Spinach (½ cup) steamed with garlic & drizzled	50	
Water with lemon wedge	10	455 Cal
SNACK		
Coffee or tea	10	10 Cal
		1200 Cal

Day 19   1200 Calorie Meal Plan

BREAKFAST	Calories	Totals
Grapefruit (½)	75	
Scrambled egg	80	
Whole-grain toast (1 slice)	70	
Coffee	10	235 Cal
SNACK		
Yogurt (6 oz nonfat, any flavor)	90	
Coffee or tea	10	100 Cal
LUNCH		
Soup (Appendix B - page 208)	90	
Small whole-grain roll	80	
Cucumber + tomato slices & 1 tsp low-cal dressing	30	
Hot or iced tea	10	210 Cal
SNACK		
Coffee or tea	10	10 Cal
DINNER		
Eat Out – Pasta dinner (Day 19 Recipe - page 131)		
Max allowable calories	640	640 Cal
SNACK		
Coffee or tea	10	10 Cal
		1205 Cal

Day 20   1200 Calorie Meal Plan

BREAKFAST	Calories	Totals
Cantaloupe (½ medium)	50	
Wheaties (¾ cup) + ½ cup skim milk + ½ banana	190	
Coffee	10	250 Cal
SNACK		
Fresh fruit in season (apple, plum, etc)	70	
Coffee or tea	10	80 Cal
LUNCH		
Peanut butter (2 Tbsp) on 2 slices of bread	340	
Hot or iced tea	10	350 Cal
SNACK		
Coffee or tea	10	10 Cal
DINNER		
Beans & Greens Salad (Day 20 Recipe - page 132)	260	
Whole-grain bread (1 slice)	70	
Baked potato (medium)	100	
Fresh fruit in season (apple, plum, etc)	70	
Water	0	500 Cal
SNACK		
Coffee or tea	10	10 Cal
		1200 Cal

Day 21 1200 Calorie Meal Plan

BREAKFAST	Calories	Totals
Cantaloupe (½ medium)	50	
Oatmeal (½ cup dry) + ½ cup skim milk + about 15 raisins	220	
Coffee	10	280 Cal
SNACK		
Coffee or tea	10	10 Cal
LUNCH		
Subway 6" (Veggie DeLite)*	190	
Fresh fruit in season (peach, plum, etc)	70	
Diet soda or water	0	260 Cal
SNACK		
Yogurt (6 oz nonfat, any flavor)	90	
Coffee or tea	10	100 Cal
DINNER		
Frozen Pasta dinner (Day 21 Recipe - page 133)	300	
Large tossed salad with 1½ Tbsp low-cal dressing	70	
Whole-grain bread (1 slice)	70	
Water with lemon wedge	10	450 Cal
SNACK		
Nature Valley Crunchy Granola bar	90	
Coffee or tea	10	100 Cal
		1200 Cal

Day 22   1200 Calorie Meal Plan

BREAKFAST	Calories	Totals
Fresh or frozen strawberries (1 cup)	25	
French toasted **English Muffin** (Day 3a Recipe - page112)	270	
Light syrup (1 Tbsp)	30	
Coffee	10	335 Cal
SNACK		
Coffee or tea	10	10 Cal
LUNCH		
Soup (Appendix B - page 208)	100	
Egg salad (1 hard-boiled egg + 1 Tbsp light mayo)	125	
Small whole-grain roll	80	
Hot or iced tea	10	315 Cal
SNACK		
Coffee or tea	10	10 Cal
DINNER		
Tomato Risotto salad (Day 22 Recipe - page 134)	370	
Whole-grain bread (1 slice)	70	
Fresh fruit in season (apple, peach, etc)	70	
Water with lemon wedge	10	520 Cal
SNACK		
Coffee or tea	10	10 Cal
		1200 Cal

Day 23 1200 Calorie Meal Plan

BREAKFAST	Calories	Totals
Tomato juice (½ cup)	20	
Shredded Wheat (1 cup) + ½ cup skim milk + ½ banana	260	
Coffee	10	290 Cal
SNACK		
Handful unsalted mixed nuts	100	
Coffee or tea	10	110 Cal
LUNCH		
Salad - 3 oz canned tuna, 1 tsp Evoo, onions & celery	175	
Small whole-grain roll	80	
Hot or iced tea	10	265 Cal
SNACK		
Coffee or tea	10	10 Cal
DINNER		
Spaghetti alla Puttanesca (Day 23 Recipe -page 135)	345	
Large tossed salad with 1½ Tbsp low-cal dressing	70	
Italian or French bread (1 slice)	80	
Water with lemon wedge	10	505 Cal
SNACK		
Coffee or tea	10	10 Cal
		1190 Cal

Day 24 1200 Calorie Meal Plan

BREAKFAST	Calories	Totals
Fresh orange sliced	75	
Soft-boiled egg	80	
Whole grain toast (1 slice)	70	
Coffee	10	235 Cal
SNACK		
Yogurt (6 oz nonfat, any flavor)	90	
Coffee or tea	10	100 Cal
LUNCH		
Salad – 3 oz canned salmon, 1 tsp Evoo, onions & celery	200	
Lettuce & tomato wedges	20	
Rye bread (1 slice)	70	
Coffee or tea	10	300 Cal
SNACK		
Fresh fruit in season (peach, plum, etc)	70	
Coffee or tea	10	80 Cal
DINNER		
Four bean salad (1 cup) (Day 24 Recipe - page 136)	270	
Large tossed salad with 1½ Tbsp low-cal dressing	70	
Water with lemon wedge	10	350 Cal
SNACK		
Graham crackers (4 squares)	120	
Coffee or tea	10	130 Cal
		1195 Cal

Day 25 1200 Calorie Meal Plan

BREAKFAST	Calories	Totals
Grapefruit (½)	75	
Cheerios (1 cup) + ½ cup skim milk + about 15 raisins	190	
Coffee	10	275 Cal
SNACK		
Fresh fruit in season (apple, peach, etc)	70	70 Cal
LUNCH		
Cottage cheese (1 cup low fat)	180	
Large tossed salad with 1½ Tbsp low-cal dressing	70	
Small whole-grain roll	80	
Hot or iced tea	10	340 Cal
SNACK		
Yogurt (6 oz nonfat, any flavor)	90	
Coffee or tea	10	100 Cal
DINNER		
Tofu w veggies & peanuts (Day 25 Recipe - page 137)	320	
Small whole-grain roll	80	
Water with lemon wedge	10	410 Cal
SNACK		
Coffee or tea	10	10 Cal
		1205 Cal

Day 26   1200 Calorie Meal Plan

BREAKFAST	Calories	Totals
Cantaloupe (½ medium)	50	
Fried eggs (2 eggs)	160	
Toasted whole-grain bread (1 slice)	70	
Coffee	10	290 Cal
SNACK		
Yogurt (6 oz nonfat, any flavor)	90	
Coffee or tea	10	100 Cal
LUNCH		
Soup (Appendix B - page 208)	150	
Hard whole-grain roll (medium)	80	
Lettuce & tomato slices	20	
Hot or iced tea	10	260 Cal
SNACK		
Fresh fruit in season (apple, peach, etc)	70	
Coffee or tea	10	80 Cal
DINNER		
Grilled scallops (Day 26 Recipe - page 138)	210	
Grilled polenta (Day 26 Recipe)	125	
Mushroom-steamed green beans-red onion	45	
Grilled asparagus	10	
Large tossed salad with 1½ Tbsp low-cal dressing	70	
Water	0	460 Cal
SNACK		
Coffee or tea	10	10 Cal
		1200 Cal

Day 27   1200 Calorie Meal Plan

BREAKFAST	Calories	Totals
Orange juice (½ cup)	50	
Oatmeal (½ cup dry) + ½ cup skim milk + about 15 raisins	220	
Coffee	10	280 Cal
SNACK		
Coffee or tea	10	10 Cal
LUNCH		
Two servings (1 cup) left over Day 24 bean salad	270	
Small whole-grain roll	80	
Lettuce & tomato slices	20	
Hot or iced tea	10	380 Cal
SNACK		
Fresh fruit in season (apple, plum, etc)	70	
Coffee or tea	10	80 Cal
DINNER		
Fettuccine (Day 27 Recipe - page 139)	290	
Large tossed salad with 1½ Tbsp low-cal dressing	70	
Italian or French bread (1 slice)	80	
Water	0	440 Cal
SNACK		
Coffee or tea	10	10 Cal
		1200 Cal

Day 28 1200 Calorie Meal Plan

BREAKFAST	Calories	Totals
Cantaloupe (½ medium)	50	
Smoothie (Day 14a Recipe - page 125)	220	
Coffee	10	280 Cal
SNACK		
Fresh fruit in season (peach, plum, etc)	70	70 Cal
LUNCH		
Grilled Swiss cheese sandwich (2 oz low-fat cheese)	320	
Cucumber + tomato slices & 1 tsp low-cal dressing	30	
Hot or iced tea	10	360 Cal
SNACK		
Coffee or tea	10	10 Cal
DINNER		
Frozen Tofu-based dinner (Day 28 Recipe - page 140)	340	
Large tossed salad with 1½ Tbsp low-cal dressing	70	
Whole-grain bread (1 slice)	70	
Water	0	480 Cal
SNACK		
Coffee or tea	10	10 Cal
		1210 Cal

Day 29   1200 Calorie Meal Plan

BREAKFAST	Calories	Totals
Cantaloupe (½ medium)	50	
Wheaties (¾ cup) + ½ cup skim milk + ½ banana	190	
Coffee	10	250 Cal
SNACK		
Fresh fruit in season (apple, plum, etc)	70	
Coffee or tea	10	80 Cal
LUNCH		
Soup (Appendix B - page 208)	160	
Small whole-grain roll	80	
Water with lemon wedge	10	250 Cal
SNACK		
Handful unsalted mixed nuts	100	
Coffee or tea	10	110 Cal
DINNER		
Tina's Healthy Frittata (Day 29 Recipe - page 141)	320	
Large tossed salad with 1½ Tbsp low-cal dressing	70	
Small whole-grain roll	80	
Water with lemon wedge	10	500 Cal
SNACK		
Coffee or tea	10	10 Cal
		1200 Cal

Day 30 1200 Calorie Meal Plan

BREAKFAST	Calories	Totals
Fresh orange sliced	75	
Kashi GoLean (1 cup) + ½ cup skim milk + ½ banana	235	
Coffee	10	320 Cal
SNACK		
Fresh fruit in season (apple, plum, etc)	70	
Coffee or tea	10	80 Cal
LUNCH		
Soup (Appendix B - page 208)	140	
Small whole-grain roll	80	
Raw zucchini slices, celery and carrot sticks	20	
Water with lemon wedge	10	250 Cal
SNACK		
Coffee or tea	10	10 Cal
DINNER		
Portobello mushroom burger (Day 30 Recipe - page 142)	270	
Lettuce and sliced tomato	20	
Whole-grain hard roll	140	
Steamed green beans	25	
Pickle spear	0	
Water with lemon wedge	10	465 Cal
SNACK		
Graham crackers (2 squares)	60	
Coffee or tea	10	70 Cal
		1195 Cal

Day 31   1200 Calorie Meal Plan

BREAKFAST	Calories	Totals
Grapefruit (½)	75	
Scrambled egg	80	
Whole grain toast (1 slice)	70	
Coffee	10	235 Cal
SNACK		
Yogurt (6 oz nonfat, any flavor)	90	90 Cal
LUNCH		
Peanut butter (2 Tbsp) 2 slices whole-grain bread	340	
Diet soda or water	0	340 Cal
SNACK		
Fresh fruit in season (pear, peach, etc)	70	70 Cal
DINNER		
Baked Sea Bass (Day 31 Recipe - page 143)	395	
Large tossed salad with 1½ Tbsp low-cal dressing	70	
Water	0	465 Cal
SNACK		
Coffee or tea	10	10 Cal
		1210 Cal

Day 32   1200 Calorie Meal Plan

BREAKFAST	Calories	Totals
Grapefruit (½)	75	
Cheerios (1 cup) + ½ cup skim milk + about 15 raisins	190	
Coffee	10	275 Cal
SNACK		
Coffee or tea	10	10 Cal
LUNCH		
Cottage cheese (1 cup low fat)	180	
Tossed salad with 1½ Tbsp low-cal dressing	70	
Small whole-grain roll	80	
Hot or iced tea	10	340 Cal
SNACK		
Handful unsalted mixed nuts	100	100 Cal
DINNER		
Fish with Orzo (Day 32 Recipe - page 144)	400	
Swiss Chard (steamed & drizzled with 1 tsp Evoo)	70	
Water	0	470 Cal
SNACK		
Coffee or tea	10	10 Cal
		1205 Cal

Day 33   1200 Calorie Meal Plan

BREAKFAST	Calories	Totals
Cantaloupe (½ medium)	50	
Fried egg	80	
Toasted raisin bread (1 slice)	75	
Coffee	10	215 Cal
SNACK		
Yogurt (6 oz nonfat, any flavor)	90	90 Cal
LUNCH		
Subway 6" (Veggie DeLite)	190	
Lettuce and sliced tomato with 1 Tbsp low-cal	45	
Diet soda or water	0	235 Cal
SNACK		
Coffee or tea	10	10 Cal
DINNER		
Frozen Vegetarian dinner (Day 33 Recipe-page 145)	340	
Large tossed salad with 1½ Tbsp low-cal dressing	70	
Whole-grain bread (1 slice)	70	
Fresh fruit in season (peach, plum, etc)	70	
Water	0	550 Cal
SNACK		
Graham crackers (3 squares)	90	
Coffee or tea	10	100 Cal
		1200 Cal

Day 34   1200 Calorie Meal Plan

BREAKFAST	Calories	Totals
Tomato juice (½ cup)	20	
Shredded Wheat (1 cup) + ½ cup skim milk + ½ banana	265	
Coffee	10	295 Cal
SNACK		
Coffee or tea	10	10 Cal
LUNCH		
Salad – 3 oz canned salmon, 1 tsp Evoo, onions & celery	200	
Lettuce & tomato wedges	20	
Rye bread (1 slice)	70	
Coffee or tea	10	300 Cal
SNACK		
Carrot sticks + ¼ cup low-fat cottage cheese & chives	60	
Coffee or tea	10	70 Cal
DINNER		
Pasta Rapini (Day 34 Recipe - page 146)	290	
Large tossed green salad with 1½ Tbsp low-cal	70	
Italian or French bread (1 slice)	80	
Water	0	440 Cal
SNACK		
Fresh fruit in season (apple, peach, etc)	70	
Coffee or tea	10	80 Cal
		1195 Cal

Day 35   1200 Calorie Meal Plan

BREAKFAST	Calories	Totals
Cantaloupe (½ medium)	50	
Oatmeal (½ cup dry) + ½ cup skim milk + about 15 raisins	220	
Coffee	10	280 Cal
SNACK		
Fresh fruit in season (apple, plum, etc)	70	70 Cal
LUNCH		
Grilled cheese sandwich (2 slices 2% cheese)	240	
Pickle spear	0	
Water	0	240 Cal
SNACK		
Carrot sticks + ¼ cup low-fat cottage cheese & chives	60	
Coffee or tea	10	70 Cal
DINNER		
Eat Out – Vegetarian restaurant (Day 35 Recipe - page147)		
Max allowable calories	530	530 Cal
SNACK		
Coffee or tea	10	10 Cal
		1200 Cal

Day 36   1200 Calorie Meal Plan

BREAKFAST	Calories	Totals
Cantaloupe (½ medium)	50	
Wheaties (¾ cup) + ½ cup skim milk + ½ banana	190	
Coffee	10	250 Cal
SNACK		
Fresh fruit in season (apple, pear, etc)	70	
Coffee or tea	10	80 Cal
LUNCH		
Soup (Appendix B - page 208)	130	
Open-face grilled cheese sandwich (1 slice 2% cheese)	120	
Water	0	250 Cal
SNACK		
Coffee or tea	10	10 Cal
DINNER		
Grilled Tilapia (Day 36 Recipe - page 148)	300	
Asparagus spears (6)	25	
Wild rice (½ cup – after cooking)	100	
Large tossed salad with 1½ Tbsp low-cal dressing	70	
Water	0	495 Cal
SNACK		
Popcorn Mini Bag	100	
Coffee or tea	10	110 Cal
		1195 Cal

Day 37 1200 Calorie Meal Plan

BREAKFAST	Calories	Totals
Orange juice (½ cup)	50	
Soft-boiled egg	80	
Whole grain toast (1 slice)	70	
Coffee	10	210 Cal
SNACK		
Yogurt (6 oz nonfat, any flavor)	90	
Coffee or tea	10	100 Cal
LUNCH		
Salad (3 oz canned tuna, 1 tsp Evoo, onions, celery)	175	
Lettuce & tomato wedges + rye bread (1 slice)	90	
Fresh fruit in season – (apple, pear, etc)	70	
Coffee or tea	10	345 Cal
SNACK		
Handful unsalted mixed nuts	100	
Coffee or tea	10	110 Cal
DINNER		
Bulgur & veggies (Day 37 Recipe - page 149)	270	
Small whole-grain roll	80	
Water with lemon wedge	10	360 Cal
SNACK		
Graham crackers (2 squares)	60	
Coffee or tea	10	70 Cal
		1195 Cal

Day 38   1200 Calorie Meal Plan

BREAKFAST	Calories	Totals
Cantaloupe (½ medium)	50	
Smoothie (Day 14a Recipe - page 125)	220	
Coffee	10	280 Cal
SNACK		
Coffee or tea	10	10 Cal
LUNCH		
Peanut butter (2 Tbsp) 2 slices bread	340	
Skim milk (4 oz)	45	385 Cal
SNACK		
Fresh fruit in season (apple, plum, etc)	70	
Coffee or tea	10	80 Cal
DINNER		
Risotto primavera (Day 38 Recipe - page 150)	365	
Water with lemon wedge	10	375 Cal
SNACK		
Graham crackers (2 squares)	60	
Coffee or tea	10	70 Cal
		1200 Cal

56

Day 39 1200 Calorie Meal Plan

BREAKFAST	Calories	Totals
Fresh sliced orange	75	
Cheerios (1 cup) + ½ cup skim milk + about 15 raisins	190	
Coffee	10	275 Cal
SNACK		
Fresh fruit in season (peach, plum, etc)	70	
Coffee or tea	10	80 Cal
LUNCH		
Cottage cheese (1 cup low fat)	180	
Large tossed salad with 1½ Tbsp low-cal dressing	70	
Small whole-grain roll	80	
Hot or iced tea	10	340 Cal
SNACK		
Handful unsalted mixed nuts	100	
Coffee or tea	10	110 Cal
DINNER		
Tofu steak & veggies (Day 39 Recipe - page 151)	275	
Water with lemon wedge	10	375 Cal
SNACK		
Coffee or tea	10	10 Cal
		1190 Cal

Day 40   1200 Calorie Meal Plan

BREAKFAST	Calories	Totals
Grapefruit (½)	75	
Scrambled egg	80	
Toasted raisin bread (1 slice)	75	
Coffee	10	240 Cal
SNACK		
Yogurt (6 oz nonfat, any flavor)	90	
Coffee or tea	10	100 Cal
LUNCH		
Soup (Appendix B - page 208)	160	
Whole-grain bread (1 slice)	70	
Hot or iced tea	10	240 Cal
SNACK		
Coffee or tea	10	10 Cal
DINNER		
Eat Out – Fish dinner (Day 40 Recipe - page 152)		
Max allowable calories	595	595 Cal
SNACK		
Coffee or tea	10	10 Cal
		1195 Cal

Day 41 1200 Calorie Meal Plan

BREAKFAST	Calories	Totals
Orange juice (½ cup)	50	
Shredded Wheat (1 cup) + ½ cup skim milk + ½ banana	260	
Coffee	10	320 Cal
SNACK		
Coffee or tea	10	10 Cal
LUNCH		
Egg salad (1 hard-boiled egg + 1 Tbsp light mayo)	125	
Small whole-grain roll	80	
Lettuce and sliced tomato with 1 Tbsp low-cal	45	
Hot or iced tea	10	260 Cal
SNACK		
Handful unsalted mixed nuts	100	100 Cal
DINNER		
Pasta e Fagioli (Day 41 Recipe - page 153)	300	
Large tossed salad with 1½ Tbsp low-cal dressing	70	
Italian or French bread (1 slice)	80	
Water	0	450 Cal
SNACK		
Graham crackers (2 squares)	60	
Coffee or tea	10	70 Cal
		1210 Cal

Day 42   1200 Calorie Meal Plan

BREAKFAST	Calories	Totals
Cantaloupe (½ medium)	50	
Wheaties (¾ cup) + ½ cup skim milk + ½ banana	190	
Coffee	10	250 Cal
SNACK		
Coffee or tea	10	10 Cal
LUNCH		
Grilled Swiss cheese sandwich (2 oz low-fat cheese)	310	
Pickle spear	0	
Hot or iced tea	10	320 Cal
SNACK		
Fresh fruit in season (apple, peach, etc)	70	
Coffee or tea	10	80 Cal
DINNER		
Frozen Fish dinner (Day 14b Recipe - page 126)	300	
Large tossed salad with 1½ Tbsp low-cal dressing	70	
Water with lemon wedge	10	380 Cal
SNACK		
Blueberry Muffin (Day 42 Recipe - page 154)	145	
Coffee or tea	10	155 Cal
		1195 Cal

Day 43   1200 Calorie Meal Plan

BREAKFAST	Calories	Totals
Fresh or frozen strawberries (½ cup)	25	
French toasted English Muffin (Day 3a Recipe page112)	270	
Light syrup (1 Tbsp)	30	
Coffee	10	335 Cal
SNACK		
Yogurt (6 oz nonfat, any flavor)	90	
Coffee or tea	10	100 Cal
LUNCH		
Salad (3 oz canned tuna, 1 tsp Evoo, onions, celery)	175	
Lettuce & tomato wedges	20	
Rye bread (1 slice)	70	
Coffee or tea	10	275 Cal
SNACK		
Handful unsalted mixed nuts	100	
Coffee or tea	10	110 Cal
DINNER		
Halibut and corn (Day 43 Recipe - page 155)	175	
Corn on the cob (medium)	100	
Mixed greens plus tomato salad	35	
Water	0	310 Cal
SNACK		
Graham crackers (2 squares)	60	
Coffee or tea	10	70 Cal
		1200 Cal

Day 44   1200 Calorie Meal Plan

BREAKFAST	Calories	Totals
Orange juice (½ cup)	50	
Kashi GoLean (1 cup) + ½ cup skim milk + ½ banana	235	
Coffee	10	295 Cal
SNACK		
Fresh fruit in season (apple, peach, etc)	70	
Coffee or tea	10	80 Cal
LUNCH		
Soup (Appendix B - page 208)	100	
Small whole-grain roll	80	
Hot or iced tea	10	190 Cal
SNACK		
Popcorn Mini Bag	110	
Coffee or tea	10	120 Cal
DINNER		
Baked Haddock (Day 44 Recipe - page 156)	420	
Large tossed salad with 1½ Tbsp low-cal dressing	70	
Water with lemon wedge	10	500 Cal
SNACK		
Coffee or tea	10	10 Cal
		1195 Cal

Day 45 1200 Calorie Meal Plan

BREAKFAST	Calories	Totals
Cantaloupe (½ medium)	50	
Fried egg	80	
Toasted whole-grain bread (1 slice)	70	
Coffee	10	210 Cal
SNACK		
Yogurt (6 oz nonfat, any flavor)	90	
Coffee or tea	10	100 Cal
LUNCH		
Soup (Appendix B - page 208)	160	
Lettuce & tomato sandwich (1 Tbsp light mayo)	170	
Water	0	330 Cal
SNACK		
Coffee or tea	10	10 Cal
DINNER		
Quinoa Salad w Veggies (Day 45 Recipe - page 157)	240	
Small whole-grain roll	80	
Water with lemon wedge	10	400 Cal
SNACK		
Blueberry muffin	145	
Coffee or tea	10	155 Cal
		1205 Cal

Day 46 1200 Calorie Meal Plan

BREAKFAST	Calories	Totals
Grapefruit (½)	75	
Cheerios (1 cup) + ½ cup skim milk + about 15 raisins	190	
Coffee	10	275 Cal
SNACK		
Coffee or tea	10	10 Cal
LUNCH		
Cottage cheese (1 cup low fat)	180	
Large tossed salad with 1½ Tbsp low-cal dressing	70	
Hot or iced tea	10	260 Cal
SNACK		
Coffee or tea	10	10 Cal
DINNER		
Poached Cod (Day 46 Recipe - page 158)	275	
Grilled potatoes	100	
Grilled cherry tomatoes	45	
Spinach (½ cup) steamed with garlic & drizzled	50	
Water with lemon wedge	10	480 Cal
SNACK		
Blueberry muffin	145	
Coffee or tea	10	155 Cal
		1190 Cal

64

Day 47 1200 Calorie Meal Plan

BREAKFAST	Calories	Totals
Cantaloupe (½ medium)	50	
Smoothie (Day 14a Recipe - page 125)	220	
Coffee	10	280 Cal
SNACK		
Coffee or tea	10	10 Cal
LUNCH		
Salad – 3 oz canned salmon, 1 tsp Evoo, onions & celery	200	
Small whole-grain roll	80	
Lettuce	0	
Hot or iced tea	10	290 Cal
SNACK		
Coffee or tea	10	10 Cal
DINNER		
Pasta Salad (Day 47 Recipe - page 159)	370	
Italian or French bread (1 slice)	80	
Water with lemon wedge	10	460 Cal
SNACK		
Blueberry muffin	145	
Coffee or tea	10	155 Cal
		1205 Cal

Day 48 1200 Calorie Meal Plan

BREAKFAST	Calories	Totals
Cantaloupe (½ medium)	50	
Scrambled egg	80	
Whole-grain toast (1 slice)	70	
Coffee	10	210 Cal
SNACK		
Yogurt (6 oz nonfat, any flavor)	90	
Coffee or tea	10	100 Cal
LUNCH		
Subway 6" (Veggie DeLite)	190	
Small bunch of grapes	50	
Diet soda or water	0	240 Cal
SNACK		
Handful unsalted mixed nuts	100	
Coffee or tea	10	110 Cal
DINNER		
Eat Out – Vegetarian (Day 48 Recipe - page 160)		
Max allowable calories	530	530 Cal
SNACK		
Coffee or tea	10	10 Cal
		1200 Cal

Day 49 1200 Calorie Meal Plan

BREAKFAST	Calories	Totals
Cantaloupe (½ medium)	50	
Oatmeal (½ cup dry) + ½ cup skim milk + about 15 raisins	220	
Coffee	10	280 Cal
SNACK		
Coffee or tea	10	10 Cal
LUNCH		
Salad (3 oz canned tuna, 1 tsp Evoo, onions, celery)	175	
Lettuce & tomato wedges	20	
Rye bread (1 slice)	70	
Coffee or tea	10	295 Cal
SNACK		
Fresh fruit in season (apple, plum, etc)	70	
Coffee or tea	10	80 Cal
DINNER		
Frozen Pasta dinner (Day 49 Recipe - page 161)	300	
Large tossed salad with 1½ Tbsp low-cal dressing	70	
Water with lemon wedge	10	380 Cal
SNACK		
Blueberry muffin	145	
Coffee or tea	10	155 Cal
		1200 Cal

Day 50 1200 Calorie Meal Plan

BREAKFAST	Calories	Totals
Fresh or frozen strawberries (1 cup)	25	
French toasted English Muffin (Day 3a Recipe page112)	270	
Light syrup (1 Tbsp)	30	
Coffee	10	335 Cal
SNACK		
Yogurt (6 oz nonfat, any flavor)	90	
Coffee or tea	10	100 Cal
LUNCH		
Soup (Appendix B - page 208)	130	
Egg salad (1 egg + 1 Tbsp light mayo)	125	
Small whole-grain roll	80	
Hot or iced tea	10	345 Cal
SNACK		
Coffee or tea	10	10 Cal
DINNER		
Pan-fried Sole (Day 50 Recipe - page 162)	325	
Large tossed salad with 1½ Tbsp low-cal dressing	70	
Hot or iced tea	10	405 Cal
SNACK		
Coffee or tea	10	10 Cal
		1205 Cal

Day 51 1200 Calorie Meal Plan

BREAKFAST	Calories	Totals
Cantaloupe (½ medium)	50	
Wheaties (¾ cup) + ½ cup skim milk + ½ banana	190	
Coffee	10	250 Cal
SNACK		
Coffee or tea	10	10 Cal
LUNCH		
Grilled cheese sandwich (2 slices 2% cheese)	240	
Lettuce and sliced tomato	20	
Canned pineapple (½ cup, no-sugar-added juice)	40	
Hot or iced tea	10	310 Cal
SNACK		
Handful unsalted mixed nuts	100	
Coffee or tea	10	110 Cal
DINNER		
Beans & Greens Salad (Day 51 Recipe - page 163)	260	
Whole-grain bread (1 slice)	70	
Baked potato (medium)	100	
Fresh fruit in season (apple, peach, etc)	70	
Water with lemon wedge	10	510 Cal
SNACK		
Coffee or tea	10	10 Cal
		1200 Cal

Day 52 1200 Calorie Meal Plan

BREAKFAST	Calories	Totals
Fresh orange sliced	75	
Soft-boiled egg	80	
Whole-grain toast (1 slice)	70	
Coffee	10	235 Cal
SNACK		
Coffee or tea	10	10 Cal
LUNCH		
Salad – 3 oz canned salmon, 1 tsp Evoo, onions & celery	200	
Lettuce & tomato wedges	20	
Rye bread (1 slice)	70	
Water	0	290 Cal
SNACK		
Fresh fruit in season (apple, plum, etc)	70	
Coffee or tea	10	80 Cal
DINNER		
Bay scallops & snow peas (Day 52 Recipe - page 164)	240	
Brown rice (½ cup – after cooking)	100	
Large tossed salad with 1½ Tbsp low-cal dressing	70	
Water with lemon wedge	10	420 Cal
SNACK		
Graham crackers (4 squares)	120	
Skim milk (4 oz)	45	165 Cal
		1200 Cal

70

Day 53 1200 Calorie Meal Plan

BREAKFAST	Calories	Totals
Grapefruit (½)	75	
Cheerios (1 cup) + ½ cup skim milk + ½ banana	210	
Coffee	10	295 Cal
SNACK		
Fresh fruit in season (peach, plum, etc)	70	
Coffee or tea	10	80 Cal
LUNCH		
Cottage cheese (1 cup low fat)	180	
Large tossed salad with 1½ Tbsp low-cal dressing	70	
Hot or iced tea	10	260 Cal
SNACK		
Handful unsalted mixed nuts	100	
Coffee or tea	10	110 Cal
DINNER		
Tofu, Bok Choy & Mushrooms (Day 53 Recipe - p 165)	330	
Brown rice (½ cup – after cooking)	100	
Water with lemon wedge	10	450 Cal
SNACK		
Coffee or tea	10	10 Cal
		1205 Cal

Day 54 1200 Calorie Meal Plan

BREAKFAST	Calories	Totals
Grapefruit (½)	75	
Cheerios (1 cup) + ½ cup skim milk + about 15 raisins	190	
Coffee	10	275 Cal
SNACK		
Coffee or tea	10	10 Cal
LUNCH		
Cottage cheese (1 cup low fat)	180	
Tossed salad with 1½ Tbsp low-cal dressing	70	
Hot or iced tea	10	260 Cal
SNACK		
Handful unsalted mixed nuts	100	100 Cal
DINNER		
Veggies with couscous (Day 54 Recipe - page 166)	310	
Small whole-grain roll	80	
Water with lemon wedge	10	400 Cal
SNACK		
Blueberry muffin	145	
Coffee or tea	10	155 Cal
		1200 Cal

Day 55 1200 Calorie Meal Plan

BREAKFAST	Calories	Totals
Cantaloupe (½ medium)	50	
Oatmeal (½ cup dry) + ½ cup skim milk +about 15 raisins	220	
Coffee	10	280 Cal
SNACK		
Coffee or tea	10	10 Cal
LUNCH		
Two servings (1 cup) left over Day 51 bean salad	270	
Small whole-grain roll	80	
Lettuce & tomato slices	20	
Hot or iced tea	10	380 Cal
SNACK		
Coffee or tea	10	10 Cal
DINNER		
Hearty Vegetable Soup (Day 55 Recipe - page 167)	360	
Large tossed salad with 1½ Tbsp low-cal dressing	70	
Italian or French bread (1 slice)	80	
Water	0	510 Cal
SNACK		
Coffee or tea	10	10 Cal
		1200 Cal

Day 56 1200 Calorie Meal Plan

BREAKFAST	Calories	Totals
Tomato juice (½ cup)	20	
Shredded Wheat (1 cup) + ½ cup skim milk + ½ banana	260	
Coffee	10	290 Cal
SNACK		
Coffee or tea	10	10 Cal
LUNCH		
Grilled Swiss cheese sandwich (2 oz low-fat cheese)	320	
Cucumber + tomato slices & 1 tsp low-cal dressing	30	
Diet soda or water	0	350 Cal
SNACK		
Carrot sticks + ¼ cup low-fat cottage cheese & chives	60	60 Cal
DINNER		
Frozen Tofu-based dinner (Day 56 Recipe - p 168)	340	
Large tossed salad with 1½ Tbsp low-cal dressing	70	
Whole-grain bread (1 slice)	70	
Water	0	480 Cal
SNACK		
Coffee or tea	10	10 Cal
		1200 Cal

Day 57 1200 Calorie Meal Plan

BREAKFAST	Calories	Totals
Cantaloupe (½ medium)	50	
Smoothie (Day 14a Recipe - page 125)	220	
Coffee	10	280 Cal
SNACK		
Coffee or tea	10	10 Cal
LUNCH		
Salad (3 oz canned tuna, 1 tsp Evoo, onions, celery)	175	
Lettuce & tomato wedges	20	
Rye bread (1 slice)	70	
Fresh fruit in season (apple, pear, etc)	70	
Coffee or tea	10	345 Cal
SNACK		
Coffee or tea	10	10 Cal
DINNER		
Salmon w Mango Salsa (Day 57 Recipe - page 169)	460	
Large tossed salad with 1½ Tbsp low-cal dressing	70	
Water with lemon wedge	10	540 Cal
SNACK		
Coffee or tea	10	10 Cal
		1195 Cal

Day 58 1200 Calorie Meal Plan

BREAKFAST	Calories	Totals
Tomato juice (½ cup)	20	
Kashi GoLean (1 cup) + ½ cup skim milk + ½ banana	235	
Coffee	10	265 Cal
SNACK		
Coffee or tea	10	10 Cal
LUNCH		
Soup (Appendix B - page 208)	120	
Cucumber + tomato slices & 1 tsp low-cal dressing	30	
Small whole-grain roll	80	
Hot or iced tea	10	240 Cal
SNACK		
Coffee or tea	10	10 Cal
DINNER		
Tofu & broccoli garlic sauce (Day 58 Recipe - p 170)	320	
Brown rice (½ cup – after cooking)	100	
Large tossed salad with 1½ Tbsp low-cal dressing	70	
Water with lemon wedge	10	500 Cal
SNACK		
Blueberry muffin	145	
Coffee or tea	10	155 Cal
		1200 Cal

Day 59 1200 Calorie Meal Plan

BREAKFAST	Calories	Totals
Grapefruit (½)	75	
Scrambled egg	80	
Whole-grain toast (1 slice)	70	
Coffee	10	235 Cal
SNACK		
Yogurt (6 oz nonfat, any flavor)	90	
Coffee or tea	10	100 Cal
LUNCH		
Soup (Appendix B - page 208)	110	
Tomato slices ¼ cup chopped fresh basil + 1 tsp Evoo	60	
Whole-grain bread (1 slice)	70	
Hot or iced tea	10	250 Cal
SNACK		
Coffee or tea	10	10 Cal
DINNER		
Eat Out – Vegetarian (Day 5 Recipe - page 115)		
Max allowable calories	595	595 Cal
SNACK		
Coffee or tea	10	10 Cal
		1200 Cal

Day 60 1200 Calorie Meal Plan

BREAKFAST	Calories	Totals
Grapefruit (½)	75	
Cheerios (1 cup) + ½ cup skim milk + about 15 raisins	190	
Coffee	10	275 Cal
SNACK		
Fresh fruit in season (peach, plum, etc)	70	
Coffee or tea	10	80 Cal
LUNCH		
Cottage cheese (1 cup low fat)	180	
Large tossed salad with 1½ Tbsp low-cal dressing	70	
Hot or iced tea	10	260 Cal
SNACK		
Handful unsalted mixed nuts	100	
Coffee or tea	10	110 Cal
DINNER		
Cashew Tofu Stir Fry (Day 60 Recipe - page 172)	275	
Brown rice (½ cup – after cooking)	100	
Small whole-grain roll	80	
Water	0	455 Cal
SNACK		
Coffee or tea	10	10 Cal
		1190 Cal

Day 61 1200 Calorie Meal Plan

BREAKFAST	Calories	Totals
Orange juice (½ cup)	50	
Wheaties (¾ cup) + ½ cup skim milk + ½ banana	190	
Coffee	10	250 Cal
SNACK		
Fresh fruit in season (pear, peach, etc)	70	70 Cal
LUNCH		
Soup (Appendix B - page 208)	90	
Lettuce & tomato sandwich (plus Tbsp light mayo)	150	
Water	0	240 Cal
SNACK		
Coffee or tea	10	10 Cal
DINNER		
Shells w Cheese & Walnuts (Day 61 Recipe - p 173)	490	
Large tossed salad with 1½ Tbsp low-cal dressing	70	
Water	0	560 Cal
SNACK		
Graham crackers (2 squares)	60	
Coffee or tea	10	70 Cal
		1200 Cal

Day 62 1200 Calorie Meal Plan

BREAKFAST	Calories	Totals
Fresh or frozen strawberries (½ cup)	25	
French toasted English Muffin (Day 3a Recipe page112)	270	
Light syrup (1 Tbsp)	30	
Coffee	10	335 Cal
SNACK		
Yogurt (6 oz – nonfat, any flavor)	90	
Coffee or tea	10	100 Cal
LUNCH		
Salad (3 oz canned tuna, 1 tsp Evoo, onions, celery)	175	
Lettuce & tomato wedges	20	
Rye bread (1 slice)	70	
Hot or iced tea	10	275 Cal
SNACK		
Fresh fruit in season (apple, pear, etc)	70	
Coffee or tea	10	80 Cal
DINNER		
Curried eggplant & tomato (Day 62 Recipe - p 174)	325	
Large tossed salad with 1½ Tbsp low-cal dressing	70	
Water with lemon wedge	10	405 Cal
SNACK		
Coffee or tea	10	10 Cal
		1205 Cal

Day 63 1200 Calorie Meal Plan

BREAKFAST	Calories	Totals
Grapefruit (½)	75	
Scrambled egg	80	
Whole grain toast (1 slice)	70	
Coffee	10	235 Cal
SNACK		
Yogurt (6 oz nonfat, any flavor)	90	90 Cal
LUNCH		
Grilled Swiss cheese sandwich (2 oz low-fat cheese)	320	
Water	0	320 Cal
SNACK		
Coffee or tea	10	10 Cal
DINNER		
Indian Shahi paneer (Day 63 Recipe - page 175)	450	
Brown rice (¼ cup – after cooking)	50	
Lettuce and sliced tomato with 1 Tbsp low-cal	45	
Water	0	545 Cal
SNACK		
Coffee or tea	10	10 Cal
		1210 Cal

Day 64 1200 Calorie Meal Plan

BREAKFAST	Calories	Totals
Cantaloupe (½ medium)	50	
Fried egg	80	
Toasted whole-grain bread (1 slice)	70	
Coffee	10	210 Cal
SNACK		
Coffee or tea	10	10 Cal
LUNCH		
Soup (Appendix B - page 208)	220	
Hard whole-grain roll (medium)	80	
Lettuce & tomato slices	20	
Water	0	320 Cal
SNACK		
Fresh fruit in season (apple, peach, etc)	70	70 Cal
DINNER		
Grilled scallops (Day 64 Recipe - page 176)	210	
Grilled polenta (Day 64 Recipe)	125	
Mushroom-steamed green beans-red onion (Day 64	45	
Grilled asparagus (Day 64 Recipe)	10	
Large tossed salad with 1½ Tbsp low-cal dressing	70	
Water	0	460 Cal
SNACK		
Graham crackers (2 squares)	60	
Skim milk (6 oz)	70	150 Cal
		1200 Cal

Day 65 1200 Calorie Meal Plan

BREAKFAST	Calories	Totals
Grapefruit (½)	75	
Smoothie (Day 14a Recipe - page 125)	220	
Coffee	10	305 Cal
SNACK		
Coffee or tea	10	10 Cal
LUNCH		
Soup (Appendix B - page 208)	130	
Small whole-grain roll	80	
Coffee or tea	10	220 Cal
SNACK		
Fresh fruit in season (apple, plum, etc)	70	
Coffee or tea	10	80 Cal
DINNER		
Frozen Vegetarian dinner (Day 5 Recipe - p 177)	340	
Large tossed salad with 1½ Tbsp low-cal dressing	70	
Whole-grain bread (1 slice)	70	
Water with lemon wedge	10	490 Cal
SNACK		
Popcorn Mini Bag	110	
Coffee or tea	10	120 Cal
		1200 Cal

Day 66 1200 Calorie Meal Plan

BREAKFAST	Calories	Totals
Tomato juice (½ cup)	20	
Shredded Wheat (1 cup) + ½ cup skim milk + ½ banana	265	
Coffee	10	295 Cal
SNACK		
Handful unsalted mixed nuts	100	
Coffee or tea	10	110 Cal
LUNCH		
Salad – 3 oz canned salmon, 1 tsp Evoo, onions & celery	200	
Small whole-grain roll	80	
Lettuce	0	
Diet soda or water	0	280 Cal
SNACK		
Coffee or tea	10	10 Cal
DINNER		
Pita Pizza (Day 66 Recipe - page 178)	430	
Large tossed salad with 1½ Tbsp low-cal dressing	70	
Water	0	500 Cal
SNACK		
Coffee or tea	10	10 Cal
		1205 Cal

Day 67 1200 Calorie Meal Plan

BREAKFAST	Calories	Totals
Cantaloupe (½ medium)	50	
Oatmeal (½ cup dry) + ½ cup skim milk	190	
Coffee	10	250 Cal
SNACK		
Coffee or tea	10	10 Cal
LUNCH		
Soup (Appendix B - page 208)	90	
Grilled cheese sandwich (2 slices 2% American	240	
Lettuce and sliced tomato	20	
Pickle spear	0	
Water	0	350 Cal
SNACK		
Carrot sticks + ¼ cup low-fat cottage cheese & chives	60	60 Cal
DINNER		
Eat Out – Fish dinner (Day 7 Recipe - page 117)		
Max allowable calories	530	530 Cal
SNACK		
Coffee or tea	10	10 Cal
		1210 Cal

Day 68 1200 Calorie Meal Plan

BREAKFAST	Calories	Totals
Cantaloupe (½ medium)	50	
Wheaties (¾ cup) + ½ cup skim milk + ½ banana	190	
Coffee	10	250 Cal
SNACK		
Coffee or tea	10	10 Cal
LUNCH		
Subway 6" (Veggie DeLite)	190	
Diet soda or water	0	190 Cal
SNACK		
Fresh fruit in season (apple, peach, etc)	70	
Coffee or tea	10	80 Cal
DINNER		
Sorba noodles & broccoli rabe (Day 68 Recipe page 180)	490	
Large tossed salad with 1½ Tbsp low-cal dressing	70	
Water	0	560 Cal
SNACK		
Popcorn Mini Bag	100	
Coffee or tea	10	110 Cal
		1200 Cal

86

Day 69 1200 Calorie Meal Plan

BREAKFAST	Calories	Totals
Orange juice (½ cup)	50	
Soft-boiled egg	80	
Whole grain toast (1 slice)	70	
Coffee	10	210 Cal
SNACK		
Yogurt (6 oz nonfat, any flavor)	90	
Coffee or tea	10	100 Cal
LUNCH		
Salad (3 oz canned tuna, 1 tsp Evoo, onions, celery)	175	
Lettuce & tomato wedges + rye bread (1 slice)	90	
Fresh fruit in season – (apple, peach, etc)	70	
Coffee or tea	10	345 Cal
SNACK		
Handful unsalted mixed nuts	100	
Coffee or tea	10	110 Cal
DINNER		
Tofu-Veggie Stir Fry (Day 69 Recipe - page 181)	230	
Small whole-grain roll	80	
Water with lemon wedge	10	320 Cal
SNACK		
100-Calorie Pack Cookies	100	
Coffee or tea	10	110 Cal
		1195 Cal

Day 70 1200 Calorie Meal Plan

BREAKFAST	Calories	Totals
Orange juice (½ cup)	50	
Wild blueberry pancakes (Day 10a Recipe - page 120)	190	
Light syrup (1½ Tbsp)	45	
Coffee	10	295 Cal
SNACK		
Coffee or tea	10	10 Cal
LUNCH		
Peanut butter (2 Tbsp) on 2 slices bread	340	
Skim milk (6 oz)	65	405 Cal
SNACK		
Fresh fruit in season (apple, peach, etc)	70	
Coffee or tea	10	80 Cal
DINNER		
Baked Cod (Day 70 Recipe - page 182)	230	
Brown rice (½ cup – after cooking)	100	
Green beans - steamed	25	
Zucchini, tomatoes & onion – steamed	45	
Water	0	400 Cal
SNACK		
Coffee or tea	10	10 Cal
		1200 Cal

Day 71 1200 Calorie Meal Plan

BREAKFAST	Calories	Totals
Fresh sliced orange	75	
Cheerios (1 cup) + ½ cup skim milk	160	
Coffee	10	245 Cal
SNACK		
Coffee or tea	10	10 Cal
LUNCH		
Cottage cheese (1 cup low fat)	180	
Large tossed salad with 1½ Tbsp low-cal dressing	70	
Small whole-grain roll	80	
Hot or iced tea	10	340 Cal
SNACK		
Coffee or tea	10	10 Cal
DINNER		
Tortellini pasta & beans (Day 71 Recipe - page 183)	450	
Water	0	450 Cal
SNACK		
Blueberry muffin	145	
Coffee or tea	10	155 Cal
		1210 Cal

Day 72 1200 Calorie Meal Plan

BREAKFAST	Calories	Totals
Orange juice (½ cup)	50	
Scrambled egg	80	
Whole-grain toast (1 slice)	70	
Coffee	10	210 Cal
SNACK		
Yogurt (6 oz nonfat, any flavor)	90	
Coffee or tea	10	100 Cal
LUNCH		
Soup (Appendix B - page 208)	150	
Whole-grain bread (1 slice)	70	
Hot or iced tea	10	230 Cal
SNACK		
Coffee or tea	10	10 Cal
DINNER		
Eat Out – Pasta dinner (Day 72 Recipe - page 184)		
Maximum allowable calories	640	640 Cal
SNACK		
Coffee or tea	10	10 Cal
		12100

Day 73 1200 Calorie Meal Plan

BREAKFAST	Calories	Totals
Cantaloupe (½ medium)	50	
Wheaties (¾ cup) + ½ cup skim milk + ½ banana	190	
Coffee	10	250 Cal
SNACK		
Coffee or tea	10	10 Cal
LUNCH		
Grilled Swiss cheese sandwich (2 oz low-fat cheese)	320	
Pickle spear	0	
Hot or iced tea	10	330 Cal
SNACK		
Fresh fruit in season (peach, plum, etc)	70	
Coffee or tea	10	80 Cal
DINNER		
Frozen Fish dinner (Day 73 Recipe - page 185)	300	
Large tossed salad with 1½ Tbsp low-cal dressing	70	
Water with lemon wedge	10	380 Cal
SNACK		
Blueberry Muffin (Day 42 Recipe - page 154)	145	
Coffee or tea	10	155 Cal
		1205 Cal

Day 74 1200 Calorie Meal Plan

BREAKFAST	Calories	Totals
Orange juice (½ cup)	50	
Shredded Wheat (1 cup) + ½ cup skim milk + ½ banana	260	
Coffee	10	320 Cal
SNACK		
Coffee or tea	10	10 Cal
LUNCH		
Salad – 3 oz canned salmon, 1 tsp Evoo, onions & celery	200	
Small whole-grain roll	80	
Lettuce	0	
Diet soda or water	0	280 Cal
SNACK		
Coffee or tea	10	10 Cal
DINNER		
Pasta Pomodoro (**Day 74 Recipe -** page 186)	420	
Large tossed salad with 1½ Tbsp low-cal dressing	70	
Italian or French bread (1 slice)	80	
Water	0	570 Cal
SNACK		
Coffee or tea	10	10 Cal
		1200 Cal

Day 75 1200 Calorie Meal Plan

BREAKFAST	Calories	Totals
Grapefruit (½ medium)	75	
Smoothie (Day 14a Recipe - page 125)	220	
Coffee	10	305 Cal
SNACK		
Handful unsalted mixed nuts	100	
Coffee or tea	10	110 Cal
LUNCH		
Salad (3 oz canned tuna, 1 tsp Evoo, onions, celery)	175	
Lettuce & tomato wedges	20	
Rye bread (1 slice)	70	
Hot or iced tea	10	275 Cal
SNACK		
Coffee or tea	10	10 Cal
DINNER		
Spaghetti squash & cheese (Day 75 Recipe - page 187)	300	
Brown rice (½ cup – after cooking)	100	
Large tossed salad with 1½ Tbsp low-cal dressing	70	
Water with lemon wedge	10	480 Cal
SNACK		
Coffee or tea	10	10 Cal
		1190 Cal

Day 76 1200 Calorie Meal Plan

BREAKFAST	Calories	Totals
Orange juice (½ cup)	50	
Kashi GoLean (1 cup) + ½ cup skim milk + ½ banana	235	
Coffee	10	295 Cal
SNACK		
Fresh fruit in season (apple, peach, etc)	70	
Coffee or tea	10	80 Cal
LUNCH		
Subway 6" (Veggie DeLite)	190	
Diet soda or water	0	190 Cal
SNACK		
Coffee or tea	10	10 Cal
DINNER		
Grilled Sea Scallops (Day 76 Recipe - page 188)	200	
Corn on the cob – one ear	100	
Tomato slices drizzled with Evoo	60	
Large tossed salad with 1½ Tbsp low-cal dressing	70	
Small whole-grain roll	80	
Water	0	510 Cal
SNACK		
Popcorn Mini Bag	110	
Coffee or tea	10	120 Cal
		1205 Cal

Day 77 1200 Calorie Meal Plan

BREAKFAST	Calories	Totals
Cantaloupe (½ medium)	50	
Fried egg	80	
Toasted raisin bread (1 slice)	75	
Coffee	10	215 Cal
SNACK		
Yogurt (6 oz nonfat, any flavor)	90	
Coffee or tea	10	100 Cal
LUNCH		
Soup (Appendix B - page 208)	150	
Lettuce & tomato sandwich (Tbsp light mayo)	180	
Cucumber slices and carrots and celery sticks	15	
Hot or iced tea	10	355 Cal
SNACK		
Fresh fruit in season (apple, peach, etc)	70	
Coffee or tea	10	80 Cal
DINNER		
Eggplant Parmesan (Day 77 Recipe - page 189)	270	
Large tossed salad with 1½ Tbsp low-cal dressing	70	
Small whole-grain roll	80	
Water with lemon wedge	10	430 Cal
SNACK		
Coffee or tea	10	10 Cal
		1190 Cal

Day 78 1200 Calorie Meal Plan

BREAKFAST	Calories	Totals
Grapefruit (½)	75	
Cheerios (1 cup) + ½ cup skim milk + about 15 raisins	190	
Coffee	10	275 Cal
SNACK		
Coffee or tea	10	10 Cal
LUNCH		
Cottage cheese (1 cup low fat)	180	
Large tossed salad with 1½ Tbsp low-cal dressing	70	
Small whole-grain roll	80	
Hot or iced tea	10	340 Cal
SNACK		
Coffee or tea	10	10 Cal
DINNER		
Trout w Lemon Capers (Day 78 Recipe - page 190)	340	
Wild rice (½ cup – after cooking)	100	
Green beans (steamed)	40	
Sautéed cherry tomatoes (Day 25 Recipe - page 137)	60	
Water with lemon wedge	10	550 Cal
SNACK		
Coffee or tea	10	10 Cal
		1195 Cal

Day 79 1200 Calorie Meal Plan

BREAKFAST	Calories	Totals
Grapefruit (½)	75	
Scrambled egg	80	
Whole-grain toast (1 slice)	70	
Coffee	10	235 Cal
SNACK		
Yogurt (6 oz nonfat, any flavor)	90	
Coffee or tea	10	100 Cal
LUNCH		
Soup (Appendix B - page 208)	130	
Small whole-grain roll	80	
Water	0	210 Cal
SNACK		
Handful unsalted mixed nuts	100	
Coffee or tea	10	110 Cal
DINNER		
Eat Out – Vegetarian (Day 79 Recipe - page 191)		
Max allowable calories	530	530 Cal
SNACK		
Coffee or tea	10	10 Cal
		1195 Cal

Day 80 1200 Calorie Meal Plan

BREAKFAST	Calories	Totals
Tomato juice (½ cup)	20	
Shredded Wheat (1 cup) + ½ cup skim milk + ½ banana	260	
Coffee	10	290 Cal
SNACK		
Coffee or tea	10	10 Cal
LUNCH		
Egg salad (1 egg + 1 Tbsp light mayo)	125	
Small whole-grain roll	80	
Lettuce and sliced tomato with 1 Tbsp low-cal	45	
Hot or iced tea	10	260 Cal
SNACK		
Coffee or tea	10	10 Cal
DINNER		
Vegetable Chili (Day 80 Recipe - page 192)	360	
Brown rice (½ cup – after cooking)	100	
Large tossed salad with 1½ Tbsp low-cal dressing	70	
Fresh fruit in season (apple, plum, etc)	70	
Water with lemon wedge	10	610 Cal
SNACK		
Coffee or tea	10	10 Cal
		1190 Cal

Day 81 1200 Calorie Meal Plan

BREAKFAST	Calories	Totals
Cantaloupe (½ medium)	50	
Oatmeal (½ cup dry) + ½ cup skim milk	190	
Coffee	10	250 Cal

SNACK		
Handful unsalted mixed nuts	100	
Coffee or tea	10	110 Cal

LUNCH		
Salad – 3 oz canned salmon, 1 tsp Evoo, onions & celery	200	
Small whole-grain roll	80	
Lettuce	0	
Diet soda or water	0	280 Cal

SNACK		
Yogurt (6 oz nonfat, any flavor)	90	
Coffee or tea	10	100 Cal

DINNER		
Frozen Pasta-based dinner (Day 81 Recipe - p 193)	300	
Large tossed salad with 1½ Tbsp low-cal dressing	70	
Whole-grain bread (1 slice)	70	
Water with lemon section	10	450 Cal

SNACK		
Coffee or tea	10	10 Cal
		1200 Cal

Day 82 1200 Calorie Meal Plan

BREAKFAST	Calories	Totals
Fresh or frozen strawberries (1 cup)	25	
French toasted English Muffin (Day 3a Recipe - p 112)	270	
Light syrup (1 Tbsp)	30	
Coffee	10	335 Cal
SNACK		
Coffee or tea	10	10 Cal
LUNCH		
Peanut butter (2 Tbsp) on 2 slices bread	340	
Skim milk (6 oz)	70	410 Cal
SNACK		
Coffee or tea	10	10 Cal
DINNER		
Avocado & rice salad (Day 82 Recipe - page 194)	410	
Hot or iced tea	10	420 Cal
SNACK		
Coffee or tea	10	10 Cal
		1195 Cal

Day 83 1200 Calorie Meal Plan

BREAKFAST	Calories	Totals
Cantaloupe (½ medium)	50	
Wheaties (¾ cup) + ½ cup skim milk + ½ banana	190	
Coffee	10	250 Cal
SNACK		
Fresh fruit in season (apple, peach, etc)	70	
Coffee or tea	10	80 Cal
LUNCH		
Grilled Swiss cheese sandwich (2 oz low-fat cheese)	320	
Pickle spear	0	
Hot or iced tea	10	330 Cal
SNACK		
Handful unsalted mixed nuts	100	
Coffee or tea	10	110 Cal
DINNER		
Lentil Soup (Day 83 Recipe - page 195)	260	
Large tossed salad with 1½ Tbsp low-cal dressing	70	
Small whole-grain roll	80	
Water with lemon wedge	10	420 Cal
SNACK		
Coffee or tea	10	10 Cal
		1200 Cal

Day 84 1200 Calorie Meal Plan

BREAKFAST	Calories	Totals
Grapefruit (½)	75	
Cheerios (1 cup) + ½ cup skim milk	160	
Coffee	10	245 Cal
SNACK		
Fresh fruit in season (apple, plum, etc)	70	
Coffee or tea	10	80 Cal
LUNCH		
Salad (3 oz canned tuna, 1 tsp Evoo, onions, celery)	175	
Lettuce & tomato wedges	20	
Rye bread (1 slice)	70	
Coffee or tea	10	275 Cal
SNACK		
Handful unsalted mixed nuts	100	
Coffee or tea	10	110 Cal
DINNER		
Black-Eyed Peas (Day 84 Recipe - page 196)	280	
Brown rice (½ cup – after cooking)	100	
Small whole-grain roll	80	
Water with lemon wedge	10	470 Cal
SNACK		
Coffee or tea	10	10 Cal
		1190 Cal

Day 85 1200 Calorie Meal Plan

BREAKFAST	Calories	Totals
Cantaloupe (½ medium)	50	
Wheaties (¾ cup) + ½ cup skim milk + ½ banana	190	
Coffee	10	250 Cal
SNACK		
Fresh fruit in season (apple, plum, etc)	70	
Coffee or tea	10	80 Cal
LUNCH		
Soup (Appendix B - page 208)	160	
Small whole-grain roll	80	
Hot or iced tea	10	250 Cal
SNACK		
Handful unsalted mixed nuts	100	
Coffee or tea	10	110 Cal
DINNER		
Tina's Healthy Frittata (Day 85 Recipe - page 197)	320	
Large tossed salad with 1½ Tbsp low-cal dressing	70	
Small whole-grain roll	80	
Water with lemon wedge	10	500 Cal
SNACK		
Coffee or tea	10	10 Cal
		1200 Cal

Day 86 1200 Calorie Meal Plan

BREAKFAST	Calories	Totals
Cantaloupe (½ medium)	50	
Fried egg	80	
Toasted whole-grain bread (1 slice)	70	
Coffee	10	210 Cal
SNACK		
Yogurt (6 oz nonfat, any flavor)	90	90 Cal
LUNCH		
Subway 6" (Veggie DeLite)	190	
Hot or iced tea	10	200 Cal
SNACK		
Handful unsalted mixed nuts	100	100 Cal
DINNER		
Tuna & Bean Salad (Day 86 Recipe - page 198)	355	
Small whole-grain roll	80	
Water	0	435 Cal
SNACK		
Blueberry muffin	145	
Coffee or tea	10	155 Cal
		1190 Cal

Day 87 1200 Calorie Meal Plan

BREAKFAST	Calories	Totals
Cantaloupe (½ medium)	50	
Smoothie (Day 14a Recipe - page 125)	220	
Coffee	10	280 Cal
SNACK		
Fresh fruit in season (peach, plum, etc)	70	
Coffee or tea	10	80 Cal
LUNCH		
Egg salad (1 hard-boiled egg + 1 Tbsp light mayo)	125	
Small whole-grain roll	80	
Hot or iced tea	10	215 Cal
SNACK		
Celery sticks + ¼ cup low-fat cottage cheese & chives	60	
Coffee or tea	10	70 Cal
DINNER		
Pasta Primavera (Day 87 Recipe - page 199)	460	
Large tossed salad with 1½ Tbsp low-cal dressing	70	
Water with lemon wedge	10	540 Cal
SNACK		
Coffee or tea	10	10 Cal
		1195 Cal

Day 88 1200 Calorie Meal Plan

BREAKFAST	Calories	Totals
Orange juice (½ cup)	50	
Shredded Wheat (1 cup) + ½ cup skim milk	210	
Coffee	10	270 Cal
SNACK		
Coffee or tea	10	10 Cal
LUNCH		
Peanut butter (2 Tbsp) 2 slices bread	340	
Hot or iced tea	10	350 Cal
SNACK		
Fresh fruit in season (peach, plum, etc)	70	
Coffee or tea	10	80 Cal
DINNER		
Frozen Tofu-based dinner (Day 88 Recipe - p 200)	340	
Large tossed salad with 1½ Tbsp low-cal dressing	70	
Whole-grain bread (1 slice)	70	
Water with lemon wedge	10	490 Cal
SNACK		
Coffee or tea	10	10 Cal
		1210 Cal

106

Day 89 1200 Calorie Meal Plan

BREAKFAST	Calories	Totals
Orange juice (½ cup)	50	
Wild blueberry pancakes (Day 10a Recipe - page 120)	190	
Light syrup (1½ Tbsp)	45	
Coffee	10	295 Cal
SNACK		
Yogurt (6 oz, nonfat, any flavor)	90	
Coffee or tea	10	100 Cal
LUNCH		
Salad (3 oz canned tuna, 1 tsp Evoo, onions, celery)	175	
Lettuce & tomato wedges	20	
Rye bread (1 slice)	70	
Water	0	265 Cal
SNACK		
Fresh fruit in season (apple, pear, etc)	70	
Coffee or tea	10	80 Cal
DINNER		
Fish stew (Day 89 Recipe - page 201)	300	
Large tossed salad with 1½ Tbsp low-cal dressing	70	
Whole-grain bread (1 slice)	70	
Water with lemon wedge	10	450 Cal
SNACK		
Coffee or tea	10	10 Cal
		1200 Cal

107

Day 90 1200 Calorie Meal Plan

BREAKFAST	Calories	Totals
Cantaloupe (½ medium)	50	
Fried egg	80	
Whole-grain toast (2 slices)	140	
Coffee	10	280 Cal
SNACK		
Yogurt (6 oz, nonfat, any flavor)	90	
Coffee or tea	10	100 Cal
LUNCH		
Soup (Appendix B - page 208)	160	
Whole-grain bread (1 slice)	70	
Hot or iced tea	10	240 Cal
SNACK		
Fresh fruit in season (apple, plum, etc)	70	
Coffee or tea	10	80 Cal
DINNER		
Crab Cakes (Day 90 Recipe - page 202)	320	
Baked potato (medium)	100	
Large tossed salad with 1½ Tbsp low-cal dressing	70	
Water	0	490 Cal
SNACK		
Coffee or tea	10	10 Cal
		1200 Cal

108

Recipes and Diet Tips

Day 1- Recipe

<u>Crumbly-Tofu Scramble</u>

16 ounces water-packed extra firm tofu
4 cups kale, chopped
3 tablespoons sesame oil
½ medium red onion, thinly sliced
1 medium red pepper, thinly sliced
1 teaspoon sea salt
1 teaspoon garlic powder
1 teaspoon cumin powder
½ teaspoon chili powder

For tofu draining and preparation tips click go to page 207. While tofu is draining, prepare sauce by adding garlic, cumin and chili powder to a small bowl and adding enough water to make a pourable sauce. Set aside.

     Warm a large skillet over medium heat. Add 2 tablespoons sesame oil, onion and red pepper. Season with a pinch of salt and pepper and stir. Cook until softened - about 5 minutes. Add kale, season with a bit more salt and pepper, and cover to steam for about 2 minutes.

     Meanwhile, unwrap tofu and use a fork to crumble into bite-sized pieces. Use a spatula to move the veggies to one side of the pan and add tofu. Sauté for 2 minutes, then add sauce, pouring it mostly over the tofu and a little over the veggies. Stir immediately, evenly distributing the sauce. Cook for another 5 to 7 minutes.

<u>Serves 4</u>. About 250 Calories per serving (not including potatoes).

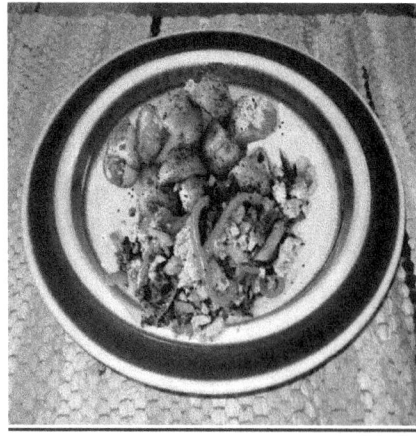

<u>Diet Tip of the Day:</u> Weight Loss – take it one step, one meal, one workout, one day at a time. Just think of where you'll be in 90 days!

110

Day 2 - Recipe

Baked Herb-Crusted Cod

4 cod fish fillets (4 to 5 ounces each)
2 tablespoons flour
2 tablespoons cornmeal
2 tablespoons minced fresh herbs
2 teaspoons lemon juice
Sprinkle cod with lemon juice. Mix flour, cornmeal and herbs and dust the cod with the cornmeal-herb mixture. Bake in oven at 375 °F for 10 minutes. Add salt and black pepper to taste.
Serves 4. One serving is about 230 Calories (for cod only).

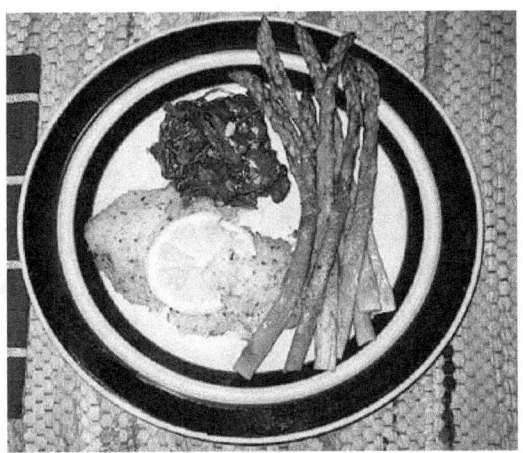

Diet Tip of the Day:. A **reducing diet is best supervised by a physician**. This is especially true when a great deal of weight needs to be lost, or if you have an ailment or a history of medical problems.

Day 3a - Recipe

French-Toasted English Muffin

6 whole wheat light English muffins, sliced in half
4 eggs
2 cups skim milk
2 teaspoons vanilla
A dash of cinnamon

In a medium bowl, beat together eggs and skim milk. Add vanilla and cinnamon. Slice English muffins into halves and saturate slices in egg mixture. In a non-stick skillet coated with cooking spray, cook muffins until both sides are golden brown. Dust lightly with confectionary sugar. Serve hot or keep in an oven or warmer at 200 °F until ready to plate. **Serves 4**. Three English muffin slices per serving. Serving is 270 Calories.

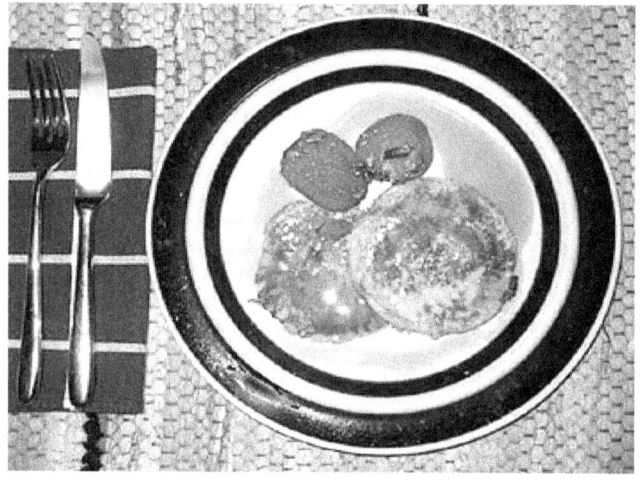

Diet Tip of the Day: **"Eat Slowly"** This is especially vital when you are trying to lose weight. If you are someone who eats fast, who finishes before everyone else at the table, you are not giving yourself a chance to feel full. While everyone else is still eating, you either sit there and pick, or you have seconds, taking in extra calories you could avoid if you would just slow down.

Polenta-Stuffed Peppers

    4 plum tomatoes, halved
    1 red onion, cut into wedges
    1 tablespoon olive oil
    4 poblano peppers, halved lengthwise and seeded
    ¼ teaspoon ground cinnamon
    ½ cup instant polenta
    1 10-ounce package frozen corn
    ¼ cup soft goat cheese (2 ounces)
    4 scallions, sliced
    kosher salt and black pepper

1. Heat broiler. On a rimmed baking sheet, toss the tomatoes, onion, and oil. Turn tomatoes cut-side down. Add the peppers, cut-side down. Broil until tender and charred, stirring the onions and turning tomatoes and peppers halfway through, 5 to 8 minutes.
2. Heat oven to 400° F. In a food processor, puree tomatoes, onion, cinnamon, ½ teaspoon salt, and ¼ teaspoon pepper until smooth. Spread half the sauce in a 9-by-13-inch baking dish. Arrange the peppers in the dish, cut-side up.
3. In a medium saucepan, bring 2¼ cups water to a boil. Add ½ teaspoon salt. Gradually whisk in polenta. Cook, whisking constantly, until thickened, 3 to 4 minutes. Stir in corn, cheese, and all but 2 tablespoons of the scallions.
4. Divide the polenta among peppers. Top with remaining sauce and bake until heated through, 5 to 10 minutes. Sprinkle with the remaining scallions before serving.

Serves 4. 290 Calories per serving

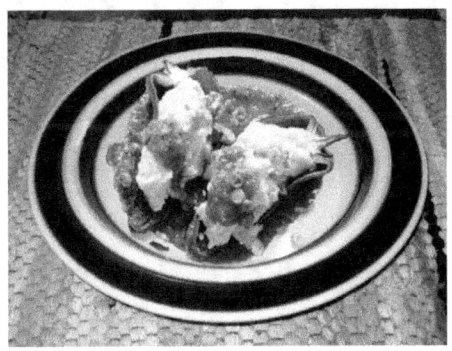

Day 4 - Recipe

Easy Penne Pasta

   1 16-ounce box whole-wheat penne pasta
   1 tablespoon olive oil
   ¼ teaspoon red pepper flakes
   1 24-ounce jar tomato-basil sauce
   ½ cup Parmesan cheese, grated
   ½ cup Italian parsley leaves, chopped

1. Bring a large pot of lightly salted water to a boil.
2. Meanwhile heat tomato-basil sauce and stir in red pepper flakes.
3. Cook the pasta according to package directions, drain and toss with tomato sauce. If desired, thin sauce with pasta water. Stir in olive oil before serving.
4. Sprinkle each serving with Parmesan cheese, parsley and salt to taste.

Serves 6.   About 375 Calories per serving

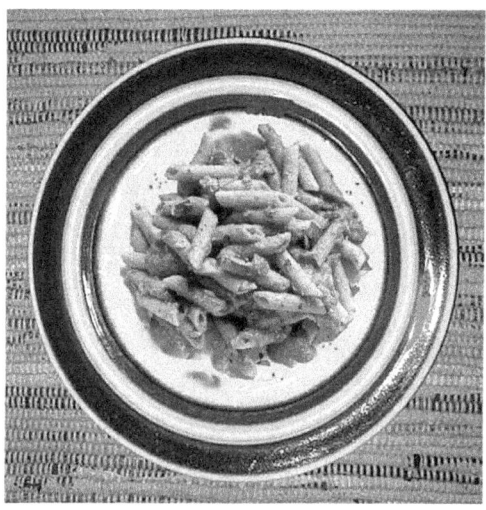

Diet Tip of the Day: **Take a daily multi-vitamin/mineral supplement.** This is very important when you're on a diet – as a kind of insurance policy.

Day 5 - Recipe

Frozen Vegetarian Dinner

No recipe today. No cooking today. It's your day off! Some reasonably good frozen vegetarian dinners are:
- Amy's Indian Vegetable Korma (310 Cal)
- Amy's Thai Stir Fry (310 Cal)
- Amy's Asian Noodle Stir Fry (300 Cal)
- Lean Cuisine Veggie Scramble (180 Cal)
- Lean Cuisine Mushroom & Spring Pea Risotto (240 Cal)
- Healthy Choice Asian Potstickers (330 Cal)

Note that if you choose any of the above entrees, you will not use all of the **340 Calories allocated for this meal**. In this case, use the excess calories anyway you wish. Splurge on extra dessert or save the calories for another day!

Please read the important **Frozen-Food Safety Warning** in **Appendix C** on page 209.

Diet Tip of the Day: **Buy a pedometer** and start walking. For the average person 2,100 steps amounts to walking about one mile. A Harvard study has shown that 8,000 to 10,000 step per day promote weight loss. And you're not obliged to walk continuously until you accrue all 10,000 steps. Rather, all steps throughout the day to wherever and whenever count toward your daily total. Because 10,000 steps a day may not be achievable by some people, particularly those who are elderly, sedentary, or who have chronic diseases, rather than insisting on a blanket 10,000 steps per day, your initial stepping goal should your baseline steps plus an increment of an additional 2,500 steps . (Your baseline being the number of steps you take in an average day.)

Day 6 - Recipe

Grandma's Pizza

The following is a pizza recipe used by Gail Johnson's Italian grandmother. She was from a small mountain village located between Rome and Naples.

Pizza dough: To save time use prepared dough, preferably whole wheat. To start, flour a large cutting board. Divide one pound of prepared pizza dough into four parts. Roll out each dough ball as thin as possible.

Tomato sauce: Sauté ½ small onion, chopped fine, in 1 teaspoon olive oil. Add two finely chopped garlic cloves, 1½ cups chopped plum tomatoes and ½ teaspoon chopped fresh oregano. Stir and cook about 5 minutes on a low flame.

Pizza preparation & cooking: On each pizza, spread evenly ¼ cup of the tomato sauce. Add ½ ounce of shredded part-skim mozzarella cheese, 1 teaspoon Parmesan cheese, 3 slices of a Portobello mushroom, some torn fresh basil, and drizzle with extra-virgin olive oil. Put pizzas on a pan and place in 475 ºF oven for about 15 to 20 minutes, or until crust is crisp and cheese is just melting. (Freeze left over sauce for use on Day 13.)

<u>Serves 4</u>. Each pizza contains approximately 350 Calories.

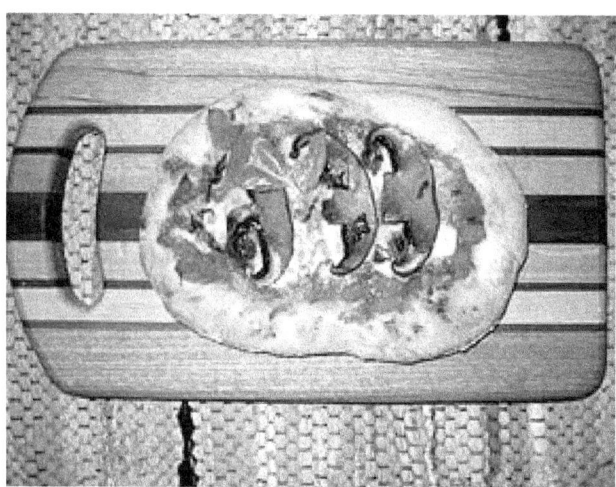

Diet Tip of the Day: For **life-long weight control** take a vigorous 30 to 60 minute walk everyday! That's right – everyday. Make exercise a nonflexible top priority part of your life. When it comes to exercise the key words are consistent, persistent, unyielding, dogged. Get the point?

Day 7 - Recipe

Vegetarian Dinner - Out

No recipe today. No cooking today. Have dinner at your favorite vegetarian restaurant, but make sure you choose a restaurant where you have a fighting chance to achieve your calorie goal. For your vegetarian dinner out, your maximum allowable calories (including appetizer, soup, main course and dessert) are as follows:

- For the **1,200 Calorie Diet**: 530 Calories
- For the **1,500 Calorie Diet**: 630 Calories

Tips for Eating Vegetarian Out: First, order simple such as tofu stir fried with vegetables, and brown rice. Tell the waiter you want little to no added sauce or gravy. Estimate the calories in the meal: tofu is about 75 Calories per ounce, most vegetable servings average approximately 50 Calories per cup, rice is about 100 Calories per ½ cup, and add about 150 Calories for the oil used in the stir fry. Then knowing your allowable calorie total for the meal, decide how much to eat – and take the remainder home. If fresh fruit is not an option, pass on dessert and have the evening snack specified for that day on this diet.

In a restaurant, most nutritionists recommend you eat the low-calorie items on your plate first. Start with the salad, soup and veggies. By the time you get to the legumes and starches you will hopefully be full enough to be content with smaller portions of the higher-calorie choices.

Incidentally, if you live in a small town with no vegetarian restaurant, to stay on this diet, have a frozen vegetarian entree. And try to abide by the allowable calorie total.

Finally, some dieticians advise their dieting clients not to eat out. That's right. They believe eating at home is safer. But our thought is you have to eat out eventually so why not learn how while your resolve is high?

Diet Tip of the Day: When you're on a diet, eating in a restaurant can be a challenge, because most restaurant portions are huge, and even a vegetarian meal can easily total more than 1,000 Calories. So, in a restaurant decide how much to eat – and take the remainder home. A good general rule of thumb is to **eat half and bring the rest home.**

Day 8 - Recipe

Baked Salmon with Salsa

This is a simple, straight-forward recipe. The advantage of a simple recipe is there are no hidden calories.

4   5 oz salmon fillets

6   tablespoons bottled tomato-pepper salsa

Brown salmon fillets in non-stick pan and then place them in a baking dish. Cook fillets in an oven preheated to 350 °F for about 10 minutes. Plate the salmon. Stir bottled tomato-pepper salsa and spoon it over the salmon.

Serves 4. One salmon fillet is about 215 Calories.

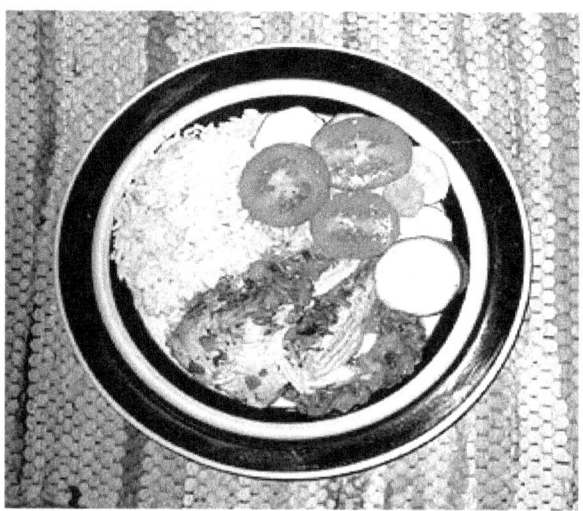

Diet Tip of the Day: Hunger is your body's way of telling you that you need calories. But **when you're done eating, you should feel better – satisfied but not stuffed**.

Day 9 - Recipe

Veggie Burger

Vegetable-based burgers can be purchased at your local supermarket. Patties of a veggie burger are made from either vegetables, soy, nuts, mushrooms, textured vegetable protein, dairy, or a combination of these foods.

In the U.S., two popular veggie burgers are the Boca Burger and Gardenburger. The Boca Burger is made chiefly from soy protein and wheat gluten. (Boca Burger patties are 2.5 oz each and range from 60 to 90 Calories.) The original Gardenburger is made from mushrooms, onions, brown rice, rolled oats, cheese, and spices. (Gardenburger patties are 2.5 oz each and about 100 Calories.)

To prepare, follow package directions. The version shown below has an added slice of low-fat cheddar cheese. The lettuce, tomato and ketchup shown actually add very few extra calories.

The veggie burger patty plus low-fat cheese amounts to approximately 150 Calories. Add a seeded roll and the total rises to 290 Calories.

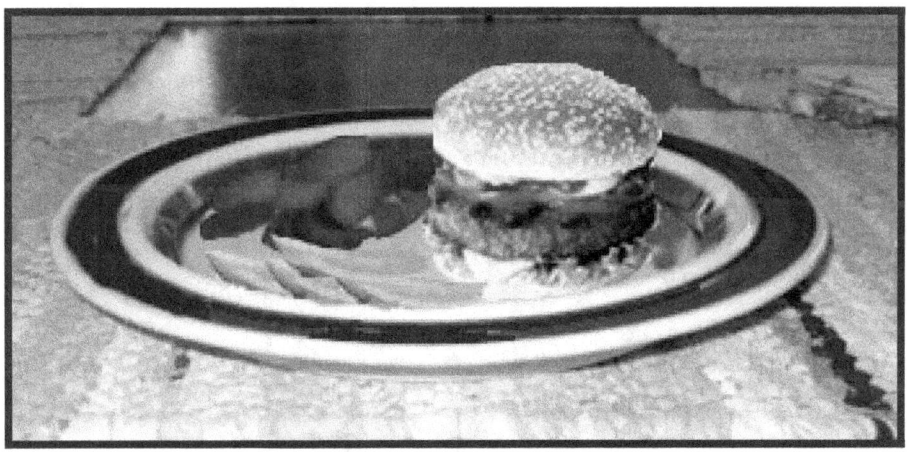

__Diet Tip of the Day:__ **Drink lots of water** – about 8 glasses per day when you're trying to lose weight. Add a slice of lemon to make it more interesting. Often, when you think you're hungry, you are just thirsty. So, next time you crave a snack, drink some water first and see if that does it for you.

Day 10a - Recipe

Wild Blueberry Pancakes

This recipe makes a relatively low calorie, wholesome batch of delicious wild blueberry-whole wheat-buttermilk pancakes.

> 1 cup whole-wheat flour
> 1 cup buttermilk
> 1 egg
> 1 tablespoon vegetable oil
> 1 teaspoon baking powder
> ½ teaspoon baking soda

Stir ingredients until blended. Add ¾ cup fresh of frozen blueberries and gently stir. Using medium heat, preheat a non-stick skillet coated with cooking spray. Pour slightly less than ¼ cup of batter onto skillet per pancake. Cook slowly until bubbles break on surface of pancake. Turn and cook until other side is lightly browned.

Makes 8 pancakes. Pictured below are three wild-blueberry pancakes with a special blueberry syrup. Sorry only two pancakes and light syrup are allowed on the 1200 Calorie diet.

Serves 4. Each pancake is about 95 Calories

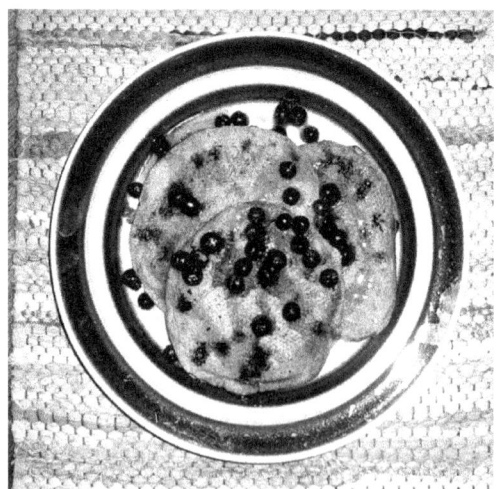

Three pancakes only allowed on 1500 Calorie diet.

Diet Tip of the Day: Most experts associate eating a substantial breakfast with successful weight loss.

Day 10b - Recipe

Lo-Cal Eggplant Parmesan

 3 medium eggplants, cut crosswise into ½-inch slices
 3 tablespoons olive oil
 1 large onion, finely chopped
 1 large clove garlic, thinly sliced
 1½ teaspoons dried oregano
 1 28-ounce can no-salt plum tomatoes or crushed tomatoes
 1 tablespoon red wine vinegar
 ½ cup (packed) fresh basil leaves
 ½ cup freshly grated Parmesan cheese
 ⅓ cup fine dry bread crumbs

1. Preheat oven to 450°F. Brush both sides of eggplant slices with olive oil, and place in a single layer on baking sheets. Bake until undersides are golden brown, 10 to 15 minutes, then turn and bake until other sides are lightly browned. Set aside. Reduce oven to 375°F.

2. Meanwhile, in a large saucepan over medium heat, add 2 tablespoons olive oil, onion, oregano and garlic. Sauté until soft, about 10 minutes. Add plum tomatoes and their juices. Break up whole tomatoes. Cover, reduce heat to low and simmer 15 to 20 minutes.

3. Add vinegar, basil and salt and pepper to taste. In a 10-by-6-inch baking pan, spoon a small amount of tomato sauce, then add a thin scattering of parmesan cheese, then a single layer of eggplant. Repeat until all ingredients are used, ending with a little sauce and a sprinkling of parmesan cheese. In a small bowl, combine bread crumbs with enough olive oil to moisten. Sprinkle on top.

4. Bake until eggplant mixture is bubbly and center is hot, 30 to 45 minutes depending on size of pan and thickness of layers. Remove from heat and allow to rest before serving.

Serves 5. About 270 Calories per serving

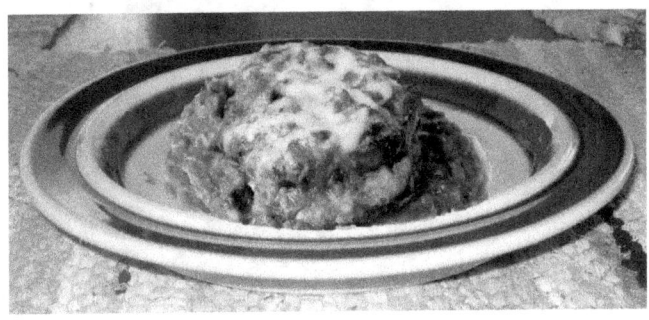

Mexican Rice and Beans

1 cup brown rice
½ small onion, diced
2 garlic cloves, minced
2 tablespoons olive oil
1 14½-ounce can diced tomatoes
1 15-ounce can black beans, rinsed and drained
1 medium fresh jalapeño, cored and finely chopped
½ cup finely chopped fresh oregano and cilantro leaves
½ teaspoon cumin, salt & pepper

1. In 1-quart saucepan, combine rice with 2 cups cold water. Bring to boil over medium-high heat, cover, reduce heat to low, and cook for 20 minutes. Remove from heat and let pan stand, covered, for another 5 minutes.

2. While rice steams, set a fine sieve over bowl and drain can of tomatoes. Pour tomato juices into a 1-cup liquid measure. Add enough water to tomato juices to equal 1 cup.

3. Heat a 10- to 12-inch skillet over medium-high heat. Pour in oil and stir-fry garlic and jalapeño until garlic browns and jalapeño smells pungent, about 1 minute. Add black beans, salt, and cumin; stir three times to incorporate mixture. Cook about 30 seconds.

4. Stir in tomato juice and water mixture and bring to a boil. Adjust heat to maintain a gentle boil and cook, stirring occasionally, until beans absorb much of liquid, about 6 minutes. Add tomatoes, oregano, cilantro, and cooked rice and cook, stirring occasionally, until rice is warm, about 2 minutes. Serve immediately.

Serves 6. About 270 Calories per serving

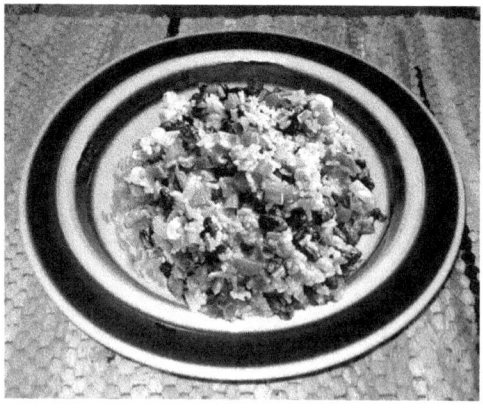

Day 12 - Recipe

Fish Dinner - Out

No recipe today. No cooking today. Have a fish dinner at your favorite restaurant, but make sure you choose a restaurant where you have a good chance to achieve your calorie goal. For today, your **goal for dinner is a maximum of 595 Calories**. This includes appetizer, soup, main course and dessert.

Tips for Eating Fish Out: First, order simple, such as broiled fish with steamed vegetables and brown rice. Tell the waiter you want no sauce, no gravy, nothing added. Then, knowing your calorie objective, and that fish is about 50 Calories per ounce, most steamed vegetable servings average approximately 50 Calories per cup, and rice is about 100 Calories per ½ cup, decide how much to eat – and take the remainder home. If fresh fruit is not an option, pass on dessert and have the evening snack specified for that day in the diet.

In a restaurant, some nutritionists recommend you eat the low-calorie items on your plate first. Start with the salad, soup and veggies. By the time you get to the fish and starches you will hopefully be full enough to be content with smaller portions of the higher-calorie choices.

Diet Tip of the Day: Phytonutrients are found in plant foods such as fruits, vegetables, whole grains, dried beans, nuts and seeds. Unlike protein, fat, vitamins and minerals, phytonutrients are not necessary for life, but evidence is growing that phytonutrients have many beneficial qualities.

Day 13 - Recipe

<u>Pasta with Marinara Sauce</u>

Prepare the sauce as you did for the Day 6 pizza (see page 116). But because the pizza sauce is a bit too thick, we add ¼ cup of pasta liquid to thin it. (The spiral pasta profile shown below is called fusilli, a very popular pasta shape because all those ridges hold buckets of tomato sauce.)

    ½ pound whole-wheat pasta
    ¼ teaspoon salt

Prepare the marinara tomato sauce as per Day 6 sauce but dilute it with ¼ cup of today's pasta liquid.

Bring 2 quarts of lightly salted water to a boil. Add pasta and stir occasionally (to keep pasta from sticking to the bottom of the pot). Keep water boiling and cook until pasta are "al dente." (Cooking time is approximately 9 minutes.) Drain pasta, add marinara sauce and serve hot.

<u>Serves 4.</u> One serving is about 225 Calories.

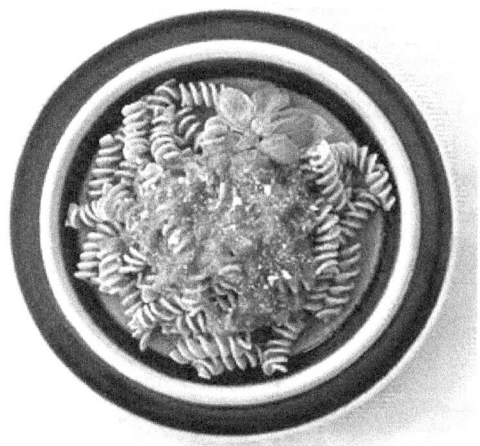

<u>Diet Tip of the Day:</u> **Beware of alcoholic beverages**. Beer has about 13 Calories per ounce, wine 25 Calories per ounce and whiskey a whopping 71 Calories per ounce.

Day 14a - Recipe

Low-Cal Smoothie

Smoothies are delicious, nutritious and fun to drink! They're great for a fast but nutritious breakfast, a light energy-boosting lunch, a healthy snack, a late afternoon pick me up, and a delicious dessert. Making your own smoothie is a smart way to save money and get healthy at the same time!

    8 ounces plain fat-free yogurt
    1 cup orange juice
    1 cup strawberries
    ½ cup blueberries
    1 banana
    1 teaspoon sugar
    1 teaspoon vanilla extract

Place yogurt, strawberries, and blueberries in a blender. Pour in orange juice. Add sugar and vanilla extract to mixture. Blend all ingredients until thick and smooth. Pour smoothie into a glass and enjoy.

Serves 2. About 220 Calories per serving

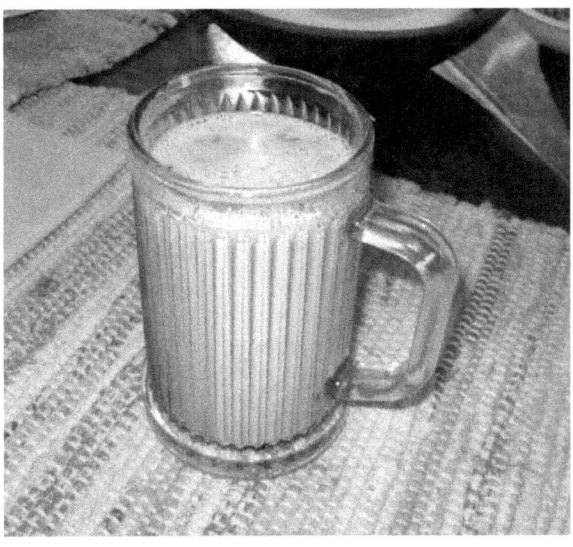

Day 14b - Recipe

Frozen-Fish Dinner

No recipe today. No cooking today. It's your day off! Some reasonably good frozen fish dinners are:
- Lean Cuisine Shrimp Alfredo (200 Cal)
- Lean Cuisine Parmesan Crusted Fish (290 Cal)
- Lean Cuisine Salmon with Basil (250 Cal)
- Healthy Choice Herb-Crusted Fish (270 Cal)

That's it. At this writing, there are just not that many frozen fish dinners for sale at supermarkets, although new entrees are being introduced continually. If you choose any of the above entrees, you will not use all of the **300 Calories allocated for this meal**. In this case, use the excess 100 or so calories anyway you wish. Splurge on extra dessert or save the calories for another day!

Please read the important **Frozen-Food Safety Warning** in **Appendix C** on page 209.

Diet Tip of the Day: Two scientific journals indicate **dark chocolate** - not white chocolate or milk chocolate - is potent antioxidant and is good for you. But don't overdo it, because you have to offset the extra chocolate calories by eating less of other foods.

Day 15 - Recipe

Spaghetti Squash & Cheese

1½-pound spaghetti squash
2 cups grape tomatoes
4 teaspoons olive oil
2 teaspoons minced garlic
4 teaspoons whole-wheat bread crumbs
1¾ cups 2% milk
½ teaspoon kosher salt
½ teaspoon freshly ground black pepper
3 ounces part-skim mozzarella cheese, shredded (about ¾ cup)
1½ ounces Parmesan cheese, grated (about ⅓ cup)
½ cup torn fresh basil leaves

1. Preheat oven to 350°F. Halve the spaghetti squash and deseed. Place both halves in a in a casserole dish (cut-side down) filled with half cup water. Cook about 45 minutes. Allow to cool 10 minutes and then scrape out spaghetti flesh with a fork into a bowl.

2. Preheat broiler to high. Combine tomatoes and 2 teaspoons of oil in a jellyroll pan. Broil 3 minutes or until tomatoes begin to break down.

3. Place a small saucepan over medium heat. Add remaining 2 teaspoons oil to pan; swirl. Add garlic; cook 1 minute, stirring frequently. Stir in flour. Add milk, salt, and black pepper, stirring with a whisk. Bring to a simmer; cook 1 minute or until thickened, stirring frequently. Remove pan from heat; stir in all but 3 tablespoons of cheeses.

4. Stir cheese mixture into the spaghetti squash then place in a small 2 quart baking dish. Stir in tomato mixture and torn basil. Sprinkle remaining cheeses over spaghetti squash mixture. Broil 2 minutes or until the top is browned. Garnish with basil leaves.

Serves 6. About 300 Calories per serving.

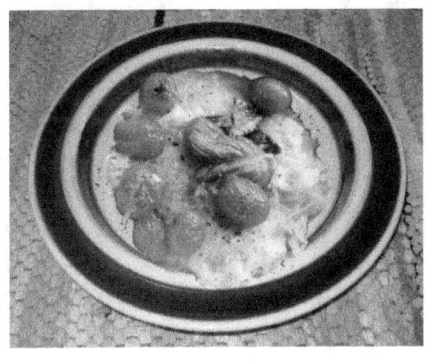

Day 16 - Recipe

Red Snapper with Special Sauce

   4 4-ounce red snapper fillets (salmon fillets okay)
   ½ cup white wine
   ½ cup non-fat yogurt mixed with ¼ cup mustard
   ½ pound green beans
   ¾ pint cherry tomatoes (about 20), halved
   4 teaspoons olive oil
   ¾ cup wild rice, brown rice and wheat berry mix.

Brown fillets in non-stick pan. Place fillets skin side down in baking dish coated with non-stick spray. Add white wine and cook in oven preheated to 350 °F for about 15 minutes . Spoon pan juices over fillets. Salt and pepper to taste.

Place green beans in skillet. Add ¼-inch of water and cook over medium heat until water boils off. Add cherry tomatoes and olive oil. Stir well and sauté for a few minutes. (If desired, season with fresh rosemary and oregano.) Salt and pepper to taste.

Prepare rice mix per package directions

Plate red snapper fillet and spoon over yogurt-mustard sauce. Add green beans and tomato mix and the wild rice mix. Serve hot.

Serves 4. One plate consisting of one snapper fillet (215 Calories) with green beans and tomato mix (75 Calories) and wild rice (160 Calories) totals 450 Calories.

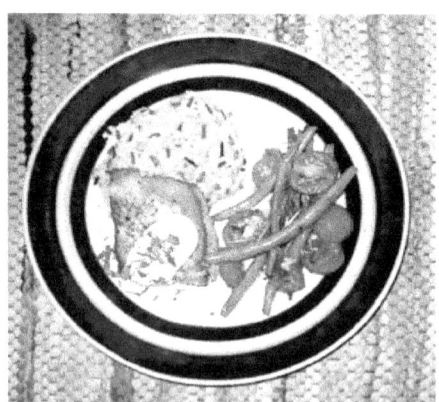

Diet Tip of the Day: **Don't have sweets in your house**. This makes them easier to resist. Out of sight, out of mind!

Vegetarian Hash

3 cups diced peeled sweet potato
2 tablespoons chopped fresh oregano
2 tablespoons olive oil
¾ teaspoon kosher salt, divided
½ teaspoon ground cumin
½ teaspoon ground cinnamon
¼ teaspoon ground red pepper
4 garlic cloves, minced
1¼ cups water, divided
1 cup green beans, trimmed and cut into 1-inch pieces
1 tablespoon adobo sauce
1 (15.5-ounce) can unsalted black beans, rinsed and drained
2 ounces soft white cheese, crumbled (about ½ cup)
¼ cup unsalted pumpkinseed kernels
1 plum tomato, seeded and diced

1. Heat a large skillet over medium-high heat. Add oil to pan; swirl. Add potato, oregano, and ½ teaspoon salt; cook 3 minutes, stirring occasionally. Add cumin, cinnamon, red pepper, and garlic; cook 1 minute.
2. Add ½ cup water; cover, reduce heat, and cook 5 minutes. Uncover; cook 2 minutes. Remove pan from heat.
3. Bring remaining ¾ cup water to a boil in a saucepan. Add remaining ¼ teaspoon salt and green beans; cook 4 minutes. Stir in adobo sauce and black beans.
4. Place ½ cup potato mixture in each of 4 shallow bowls; top each with ½ cup bean mixture, 2 tablespoons cheese, 1 tablespoon pumpkinseeds, and 1 tablespoon tomato.

Serves 4. About 320 Calories per serving

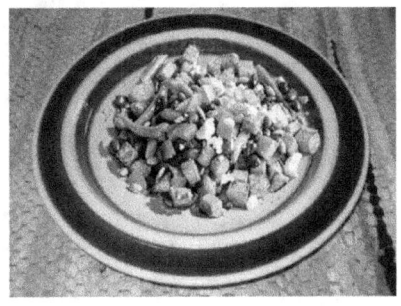

Day 18 - Recipe

Grilled Swordfish

1¼ pounds swordfish
1 bottle citrus-herb marinade
¾ pint cherry tomatoes (about 20), halved
4 medium potatoes
2 cups fresh spinach
1 teaspoon rosemary & juice of ¼ lemon
2 teaspoon extra-virgin olive oil, divided
Steam spinach with garlic and drizzle with about 1 teaspoon extra-virgin olive oil.

Cut potatoes in medium-size pieces and sprinkle with lemon juice, add rosemary, salt and black pepper. Place potatoes on grill for about 10 minutes, turning occasionally.

Toss cherry tomatoes in remaining extra-virgin olive oil. Add fresh oregano, salt and black pepper. Place on heavy-duty aluminum foil, seal and grill for about 3 minutes.

Marinade swordfish in citrus-herb vinaigrette. Grill on hot fire for about 5 minutes on one side and 3 minutes on the other, or until done as desired. **Serves 4**. One plate of grilled swordfish (250 Calories) with potatoes (100 Calories), cherry tomatoes (45 Calories) and steamed spinach (50 Calories) totals 445 Calories.

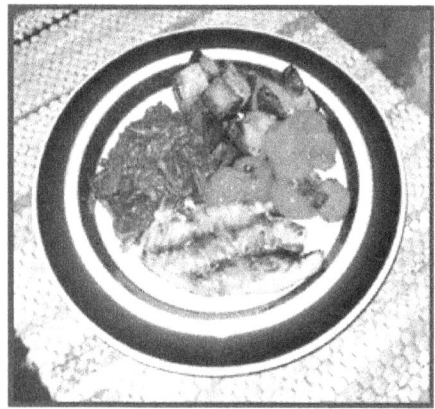

Diet Tip of the Day: **Slow weight loss is healthier**, is more likely to be permanent and is easier to sustain over the long haul. When it comes to weight loss, don't be in a hurry!

Day 19 - Recipe

Pasta-Based Dinner - Out

No recipe today. No cooking today. Have a pasta dinner at your favorite Italian restaurant, but make sure you choose a restaurant where you have a reasonable chance to achieve your calorie goal. For today, **your goal for dinner is a maximum of 640 Calories**. This includes any appetizer, soup, main course and any dessert.

Tips for Eating Pasta: Americans adore Italian food. But you can consume a lot of calories in an Italian restaurant – if you order carelessly. For example a typical portion of Fried calamari with garlic bread totals more than 1,100 Calories!

First rule, order simple. Look for pasta in a marinara sauce and a salad with dressing on the side. Then, knowing your 640 Calorie objective, and that most pastas are about 50 Calories per ounce, and marinara tomato sauce averages about 70 Calories per half cup, decide how much of the meal you can eat – and take the remainder home. To stay within your maximum allowable calorie total, you should pass on dessert and have the evening snack specified for that day in the diet.

<u>Diet Tip of the Day:</u> Another dilemma for dieters is **judging portion size**. It makes no sense to worry about whether to apportion 70 or 80 Calories per ounce for a cut of lean meat if you have no idea whether the portion you are planning to eat weighs four or ten ounces. To be successful, you must learn to estimate portion sizes with reasonable accuracy.

Day 20 - Recipe

Beans & Greens Salad

⅓ cup chopped oregano
⅓ cup chopped parsley
3 cloves garlic, chopped
1 lemon, juiced

Prepare dressing by combining above ingredients and stirring in ¼ cup extra-virgin olive oil. Salt and black pepper to taste.

½ pound mesclun mix
¼ pound green beans
19-oz can garbanzo beans (chickpeas)

Arrange mesclun mix, garbanzo beans and green beans on large platter. Drizzle dressing over beans and greens.

Serves 4. Approximately 260 Calories per serving.

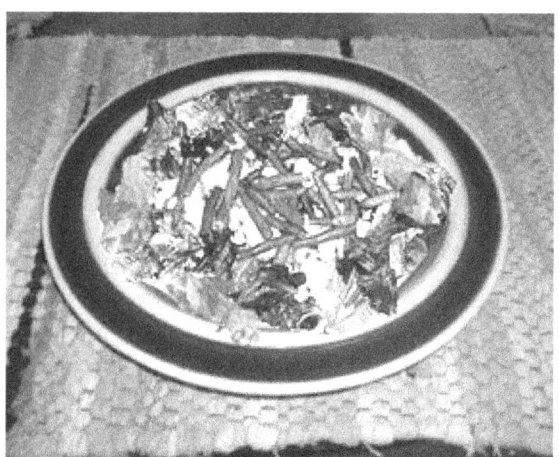

Diet Tip of the Day: Beans are a wonderful food but **beans are an incomplete protein**. If however beans are eaten with a whole-grain bread, the combination forms a complete protein – just as complete and nutritious as meat, poultry, or fish.

Day 21 - Recipe

Frozen Pasta-Based Dinner

No recipe today. No cooking today. It's your day off! Some reasonably good frozen pasta dinners are:
- Lean Cuisine Angel Hair Pomodoro (220 Cal)
- Lean Cuisine Cheese Ravioli (250 Cal)
- Healthy Choice Portobella Spinach Parmesan (230 Cal)
- Healthy Choice Portobella Marsala Pasta (230 Cal)
- Amy's Light & Lean Spagehetti Italiano (240 Cal)

If you choose any of the above entrees, you will not use all of the **300 Calories allocated for this meal**. In this case, use the excess 100 or so calories anyway you wish. Splurge on extra dessert or save the calories for another day!

Please read the important **Frozen-Food Safety Warning** in **Appendix C** on page 209.

Diet Tip of the Day: **Understanding nutrition** is not only vital for good health but also will help you control your weight over the long term. For example, did you know that foods that are labeled an "excellent source" of a particular nutrient provide 20% or more of the Recommended Daily Value. Whereas, foods that are a "good source" of a nutrient provide between 10 and 20% of the Recommended Daily Value.

Day 22 - Recipe

Tomato Risotto Salad

   1 bag microwave-in-bag green beans
   1¾ cups lower-sodium vegetable broth
   2 tablespoons butter
   1 small onion
   2 cups Arborio rice
   2 pounds ripe tomatoes
   2 cups fresh corn kernels
   2 ounces grated Parmesan cheese
   2 tablespoons chopped basil

1) Cook green beans according to package directions. Cut into 1-inch.
pieces.
2) In 2-quart saucepan, heat broth and 2 cups water to boiling. While
broth mixture heats, in 4-quart bowl, microwave butter and onion,
uncovered, on high for 3 minutes or until softened. Stir in rice and cook
another minute.
3) Stir broth-water mixture into rice mixture. Cover with vented plastic
wrap; microwave on medium (50% power) about 10 minutes.
4) Meanwhile, in food processor, puree half of tomatoes; strain juice
through sieve into measuring cup, pressing on solids. Discard solids and
chop remaining tomatoes. Stir 1½cups tomato juice into rice mixture.
Cover with vented plastic wrap and microwave on Medium heat 5 minutes
or until liquid is absorbed.
5) Stir corn into rice mixture. Cover with vented plastic wrap; microwave
on Medium 3 minutes or until corn is heated through. Stir Parmesan
cheese, green beans, tomatoes, half of basil, ½ teaspoon salt, and ¼
teaspoon pepper into rice mixture (the risotto). Sprinkle with basil.
Serves 6. 370 Calories per serving.

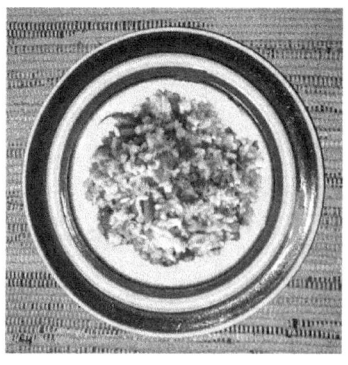

Day 23 - Recipe

Quick Pasta alla Puttanesca

This famous pasta dish originated in Naples Italy. Puttanesca means "ladies of the night." Although the exact origin of the name is unclear, one thing is clear: It's delicious! Here is one of many recipe versions.

½ pound spaghetti (whole wheat preferred)
20 black or green pitted olives
14.5-oz can diced tomatoes
4 oz tomato sauce
2 tablespoon extra-virgin olive oil
3 cloves of garlic, chopped
1 tablespoon dried minced onion
½ teaspoon crushed red pepper flakes
1 tablespoon capers drained and rinsed
¼ cup currants

Cook spaghetti according to package directions. Drain and return spaghetti to pot; add a teaspoon extra-virgin olive oil and toss to coat.

Heat remaining olive oil in large skillet over medium-high heat. Add red pepper flakes; cook and stir 1 to 2 minutes or until sizzling. Add onion and garlic; cook and stir 1 minute. Add canned tomatoes with juice, tomato sauce, olives, currants and capers. Cook over medium-high heat, stirring frequently, until sauce is heated through.

Serves 4. About 345 Calories per serving

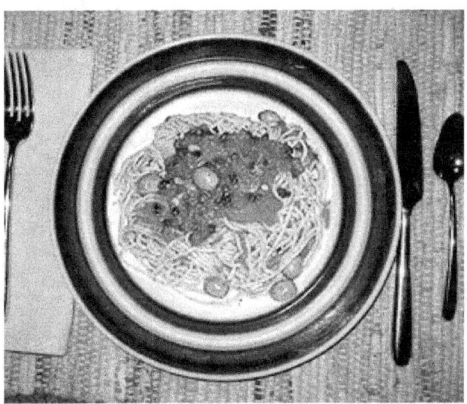

Diet Tip of the Day: Dilute fruit juices, such as apple juice, orange, etc. with water. This cuts the flavor slightly but really reduces calorie content.

Day 24- Recipe

Four-Bean Plus Salad

Note that the total caloric value of the salad will change very little, if the proportions of the bean varieties and corn are varied – according to taste.

½ cup canned red kidney beans, drained and rinsed
½ cup canned black beans, drained and rinsed
½ cup canned chick peas, drained and rinsed
½ cup canned cannelloni beans, drained and rinsed
½ cup canned corn, drained
1 small red pepper, chopped
1 small green pepper, chopped
2 tablespoons extra-virgin olive oil
2 tablespoons lemon juice

In a large bowl mix red kidney beans, black beans, chick peas, cannelloni beans, corn and chopped red and green peppers. Stir in olive oil and lemon juice and plate.

Serves about 6. One serving is ½ cup – with about 135 Calories per serving

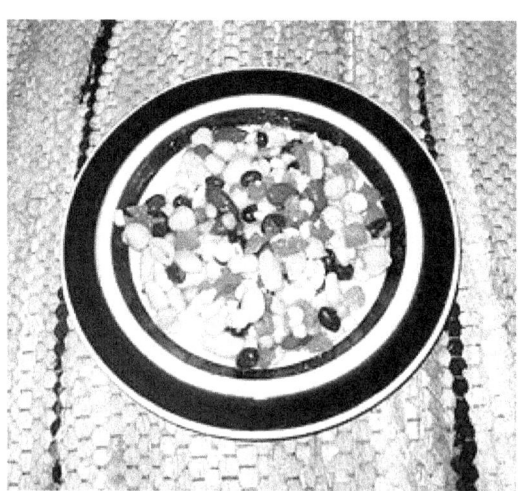

Diet Tip of the Day: Vigorous exercise doesn't necessarily stimulate you to overeat. Just the opposite. In many cases, exercise actually helps curb your appetite – immediately following a workout.

Day 25 - Recipe

Tofu with Veggies & Peanuts

2 3½-ounce bags boil-in-bag jasmine rice
1 14-ounce package water-packed firm tofu
½ cup fat-free, less-sodium vegetable broth
1 tablespoon ground fresh chili paste
1 tablespoon less-sodium soy sauce
1 teaspoon cornstarch
2 teaspoons black bean garlic sauce
1 tablespoon canola oil
1 8-ounce package pre-sliced mushrooms
1 tablespoon bottled ground fresh ginger
¼ teaspoon salt
½ cup matchstick-cut carrots
½ cup chopped green onions
¼ cup unsalted dry-roasted peanuts, chopped

1. Preheat broiler. Cook rice according to package directions, omitting salt and fat.
2. Drain tofu and cut into 1-inch pieces. (For tofu draining and preparation tips go to page 207.) Arrange tofu in a single layer on a foil-lined pan coated with cooking spray. Broil 14 minutes or until golden.
3. While tofu cooks, combine broth and next 4 ingredients (through black bean sauce), stirring with a whisk; set aside.
4. Heat oil in a large nonstick skillet over medium-high heat. Add salt and mushrooms; sauté 4 minutes or until mushrooms begin to release liquid, stirring occasionally. Stir in carrots and ginger; cook 1 minute. Add broth mixture; cook 30 seconds or until sauce begins to thicken. Remove from heat; stir in tofu and onions. Serve over rice; sprinkle with peanuts.
Serves 4. About 320 Calories per serving

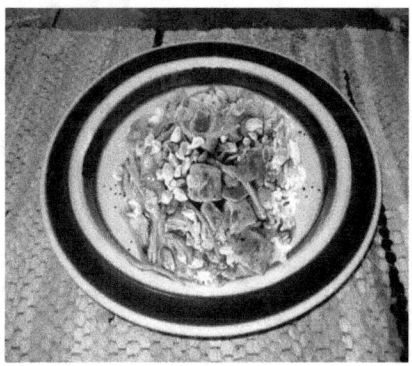

Day 26 - Recipe

Tina's Grilled Scallops & Polenta

We were going to discard this meal because some Pesceterians do not eat the scallops, but it's so delicious Gail wouldn't do it. So, please skip this meal if you don't eat scallops.

   1 pound sea scallops
   ¾ cup polenta cornmeal
   ¾ cup skim milk
   1 medium portobello mushroom
   ½ pound green beans
   ¼ cup chopped red onion
   16 asparagus spear
   1 teaspoon extra-virgin olive oil

Bring 1½ cups of water and skim milk to rapid boil. Add salt to taste and slowly add polenta while stirring. Reduce heat. Continue stirring until desired consistency is reached. Pour polenta into lightly greased pan. After polenta has cooled cover and refrigerate. Cut chilled polenta into 4 pieces. Grill on medium-hot fire – about two minutes on each side.

Brush portobello mushroom and asparagus spear with olive oil and place on grill for about 3 minutes on each side.

Grill scallops on medium-hot fire. Turn after two minutes or when first side turns opaque. Grill until second side turns opaque – about another 2 minutes. Don't overcook but test a scallop by cutting to make sure it's cooked through. Salt and pepper to taste.

Serves 4. The food on the plate pictured below totals about 380 Calories.

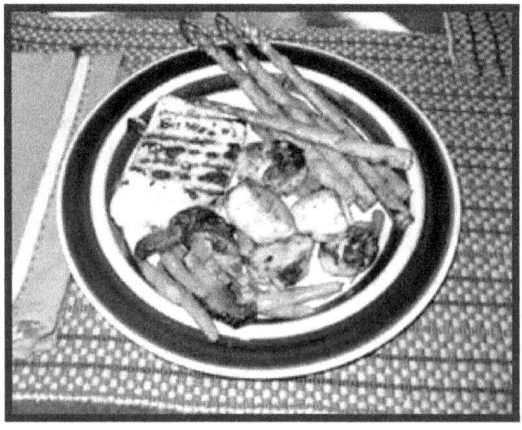

Day 27 - Recipe

Fettuccine in Summer Sauce

This sauce is often served in the summer because it's lighter than what is usually dished up with pasta. But despite its name the sauce is wonderful year round.

½ lb fettuccine
8 oz fresh asparagus, trimmed & cut in 2-inch pieces
¾ pint cherry tomatoes (about 20), halved
2 Tbsp plus 1 tsp extra-virgin olive oil, divided
2 cloves of garlic, chopped
½ small onion, diced

Cook fettuccine according to package directions. Drain and return pasta to pot; add a teaspoon of the olive oil and toss to coat. Meanwhile steam asparagus and drain.

In large skillet over medium-high heat, sauté cherry tomatoes in remaining 2 tablespoons of olive oil until skin begins to crack. Add onion and cook until translucent. Stir in garlic. Thin sauce with pasta liquid to desired consistency. Toss cooked pasta and asparagus into sauce and serve immediately.

Serves 4. About 290 Calories per serving

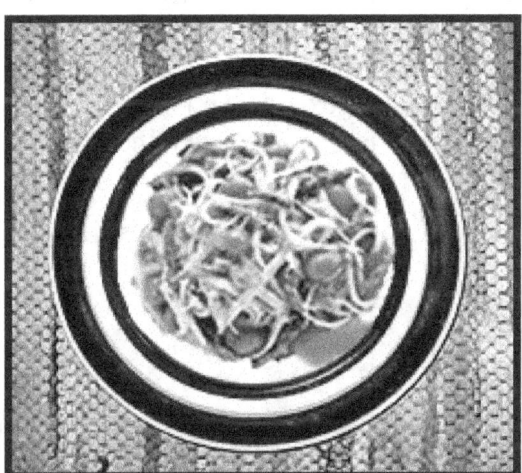

Diet Tip of the Day: A major weight-loss fallacy is that you can **get rid of abdominal fat** by working your abdominal muscles. This is based on the incorrect belief that fat is eliminated from a particular part of your body if you engage the muscles underneath that layer of fat. No such luck.

Day 28 - Recipe

Frozen Tofu-based Dinner

No recipe today. No cooking today. It's your day off! Some reasonably good frozen tofu-based dinners are:
- Amy's Tofu Scramble (320 Cal)
- Amy's Thai Stir Fry (310 Cal)
- Amy's Teriyaki Bowl (290 Cal)
- Amy's Brown Rice & Vegetables Bowl (260 Cal)

That's it. At this writing, there are just not that many frozen Tofu-based dinners for sale at supermarkets, although there could be new entrees introduced after this book "went to press." If you choose any of the above entrees, you will not use all of the **340 Calories allocated for this meal**. In this case, use the excess 100 or so calories anyway you wish. Splurge on extra dessert or save the calories for another day!

Please read the important **Frozen-Food Safety Warning** in **Appendix C** on page 209.

Diet Tip of the Day: The **general weight-change rule is "last on first off."** Assume as you gained weight, the first place you noticed it was on your thighs, next your buttocks, then your face. As you lose weight, it generally will come off in the reverse order, first from your face, then your rear and finally your thighs. And there is not much you can do about that. The truth is there is no food, no exercise, no magic belt, and no pill that will cause your body to lose fat in one place rather than another.

Day 29 - Recipe

Tina's Healthy Frittata

3 large eggs, plus 3 egg whites
¾ cup reduced-fat cottage cheese
4 ounces smoked gouda cheese, shredded (about 1 cup)
1 teaspoon minced fresh rosemary
3 cloves garlic, thinly sliced
2 tablespoons EVOO
1 medium onion, chopped
16-ounce package frozen mixed vegetables, thawed
2 tablespoons grated parmesan cheese
1 scant teaspoon paprika

Position a rack in the upper third of your oven and preheat to 450 degrees F. Whisk eggs and egg whites in a bowl. Add the cottage cheese and whisk until almost smooth. Whisk in the gouda and rosemary. In a 10-inch nonstick skillet over medium-high, cook the garlic in the olive oil. Heat until garlic starts to brown, about 1 to 2 minutes. Add onion, season with salt and cook 2 minutes. Add the vegetables, increase the heat to high and cook until just tender, about 5 minutes. Reduce the heat to medium.

Spread the egg mixture evenly in the pan. Cook, without disturbing until a thin crust forms on the bottom, about 2 minutes. Run a rubber spatula around the edge to release egg from the pan. Continue cooking until the bottom is golden, about 2 to 3 minutes. Sprinkle with the parmesan and paprika. Transfer skillet to the oven and bake about 5 to 7 minutes. Remove from the oven, cover and let sit, 5 to 7 minutes. Cut into 4 wedges.

Serves 4. 320 Calories per serving (¼ of frittata)

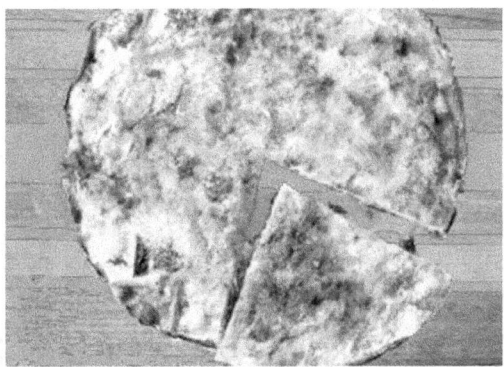

Photo shows frittata on cutting board - hot from skillet.

Day 30 - Recipe

Portobello Mushroom Burger

¼ cup low-sodium soy sauce
¼ cup balsamic vinegar
2 tablespoons olive oil
3 garlic cloves, minced
4 (4-inch) portobello mushroom caps
1 small red bell pepper
¼ cup light mayonnaise
½ teaspoon olive oil
⅛ teaspoon ground red pepper
4 (2-ounce) sandwich buns
4 (¼-inch-thick) slices tomato
4 curly leaf lettuce leaves

1. Combine first 4 ingredients in a large zip-top plastic bag; add mushrooms to bag. Seal and marinate at room temperature for 2 hours, turning bag occasionally. Remove mushrooms from bag. Start grill to medium heat.

3. Cut bell pepper in half lengthwise; discard seeds and membranes. Place pepper halves on grill rack coated with cooking spray; grill 15 minutes or until blackened, turning occasionally. Place in a zip-top plastic bag; seal. Let stand 10 minutes. Peel. Finely chop 1 pepper half; place in a small bowl. Add mayonnaise, ½ teaspoon oil, and ground red pepper; stir well.

4. Place mushrooms, gill sides down, on grill rack coated with cooking spray; grill 4 minutes on each side. Place buns, cut sides down, on grill rack coated with cooking spray; grill 30 seconds on each side or until toasted. Spread 2 tablespoons mayonnaise mixture on top half of each bun. Place 1 mushroom on bottom half of each bun. Top each mushroom with 1 tomato slice and 1 lettuce leaf.

Serves 4. About 270 Calories per serving.

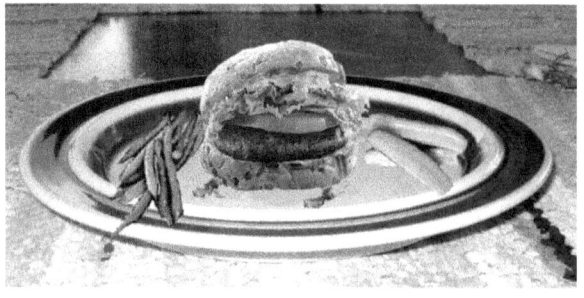

Day 31 - Recipe

Tina's Baked Sea Bass

   4 4-ounce Chilean sea bass fillets
   ½ pound green beans
   ¾ pint cherry tomatoes (about 20)
   ¾ cup brown rice (prepare per package directions)

<u>Sea Bass:</u> Dust filets with flour. Dip in egg wash & then Panko bread crumbs. Place fillets in baking dish coated with non-stick spray. Bake about 15 minutes in oven preheated to 350 °F.

<u>Green Beans & Tomato:</u> Place green beans in skillet. Add ¼-inch of water and cook over medium heat until water boils off. Add cherry tomatoes and olive oil. Stir well and sauté for a few minutes. Season with fresh rosemary and oregano.

<u>Brown Rice-Pesto mix:</u> Prepare brown rice per package directions. Add 4 teaspoons packaged "green" pesto. Mix thoroughly.

<u>Red Pepper Sauce:</u> Blend one roasted red pepper (skinned), ½ cup non-fat yogurt, 1 tsp lemon juice, 1 Tbsp olive oil, 1 Tbsp chili sauce, and a dash of Worcestershire sauce.

Serves 4. One plate consisting of one sea bass fillet with spooned over red pepper sauce (150 Calories), green beans & tomato mix (75 Calories), brown rice-pesto mix (120 Calories) and half ear of corn (50 Calories) – totals about 395 Calories.

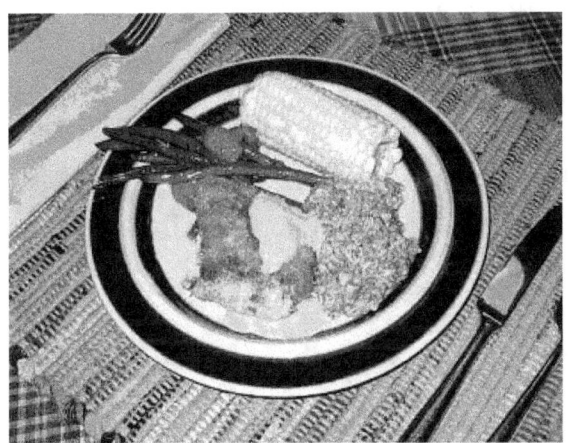

<u>Diet Tip of the Day:</u> Protein foods make you **feel full longer** and help prevent overeating.

Day 32 - Recipe

Vjay Gupta does not eat shrimp but Gail Johnson does. We were going to discard the meal because some Pesceterians do not eat the shrimp, but it's so delicious Gail wouldn't do it. So, please skip this meal if you don't eat shrimp.

Shrimp with Orzo

1 pound medium shrimp, peeled & deveined
2 tablespoons olive oil, divided
2 cloves garlic, minced
1 onion, diced
½ teaspoon dried oregano
8 ounces orzo pasta
1 pint cherry tomatoes (about 30), halved

1. Cook orzo according to package directions. After cooked, drain and return orzo to pot; add a teaspoon of the olive oil and toss to coat. Retain orzo liquid for later use.
2. In large skillet over medium-high heat, sauté cherry tomatoes in remaining olive oil until skin begins to crack. Stir in onion, garlic and oregano. Just before garlic turns slightly yellow add shrimp and sauté on both sides for 1 minute. Thin sauce with orzo liquid to desired consistency.
3. Plate shrimp and orzo and pour sauce over both. Add steamed Swiss chard. Serve immediately.

Serves 4. About 400 Calories per serving

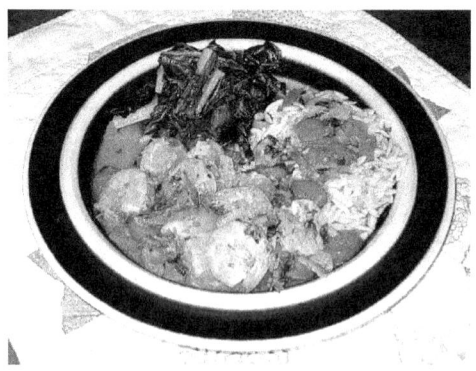

Diet Tip of the Day: It's a lot easier to eat 1,000 Calories than it is to burn 1,000 Calories exercising. Exercise is good, but a stroll after dinner isn't going to offset the calories you ingested eating a Big Mac plus fries.

Day 33 - Recipe

Frozen Vegetarian Dinner

No recipe today. No cooking today. It's your day off! Some reasonably good frozen vegetarian dinners are:
- Amy's Indian Vegetable Korma (310 Cal)
- Amy's Thai Stir Fry (310 Cal)
- Amy's Asian Noodle Stir Fry (300 Cal)
- Lean Cuisine Veggie Scramble (180 Cal)
- Lean Cuisine Mushroom & Spring Pea Risotto (240 Cal)
- Healthy Choice Asian Potstickers (330 Cal)

Note that if you choose any of the above entrees, you will not use all of the **340 Calories allocated for this meal**. In this case, use the excess 100 or so calories anyway you wish. Splurge on extra dessert or save the calories for another day!

Please read the important **Frozen-Food Safety Warning** in **Appendix C** on page 209.

Diet Tip of the Day: It's amazing how many people tend to confuse thirst with hunger. This often results in overeating when actually drinking water might be the solution. So, the next time you have a seemingly uncontrollable food craving, try drinking a glass of water instead.

Day 34 - Recipe

Pasta Rapini

    2 cloves garlic - coarsely chopped
    1½ cups of crushed San Marzano tomatoes
    2 cups Rapini (broccoli rabe)
    1 tablespoon crushed red pepper flakes (optional)
    ½ pound medium-sized whole wheat pasta

Tomato Sauce: In large pan, sauté two tablespoons olive oil over medium-high heat. Add the garlic and sauté until translucent (but not browned). Add crushed San Marzano tomatoes (use plum tomatoes if San Marzano are not available) and bring to a boil. Reduce heat to low and simmer for about 30 minutes or until cooked. Season with salt and pepper. Set aside.

Rapini: Discard the tough stems and slice into 2-inch pieces. Bring a pot of water to a boil. Add Rapini (a variety of the vegetable broccoli rabe) and 1 tablespoon salt. Blanch Rapini about 5 minutes or until slightly cooked but still crunchy at stems. Drain, set aside and cover.

Cook pasta according to package instructions until al dente. Three minutes before pasta is ready, add the Rapini to the sauté pan (containing the tomato sauce). Heat mixture over medium heat. Drain pasta and add it to the pan with the Rapini and tomatoes. Add hot pepper flakes (optional) and toss for 1 to 2 minutes over high heat. Drizzle lightly with extra virgin olive oil and plate. Delicious!
Serves 4. About 290 Calories per serving

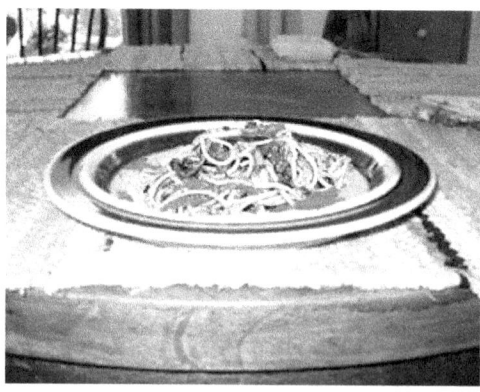

Diet Tip of the Day: Keep a daily food log to **record everything you eat**. For some people it really works wonders.

Day 35 - Recipe

Vegetarian Dinner - Out

No recipe today. No cooking today. Have dinner at your favorite vegetarian restaurant, but make sure you choose a restaurant where you have a fighting chance to achieve your calorie goal. For your vegetarian dinner out, your maximum allowable calories (including appetizer, soup, main course and dessert) are as follows:

- For the **1,200 Calorie Diet**: 530 Calories
- For the **1,500 Calorie Diet**: 630 Calories

Tips for Eating Vegetarian Out: First, order simple such as tofu stir fried with vegetables, and brown rice. Tell the waiter you want little to no added sauce or gravy. Estimate the calories in the meal: tofu is about 75 Calories per ounce, most vegetable servings average approximately 50 Calories per cup, rice is about 100 Calories per ½ cup, and add about 150 Calories for the oil used in the stir fry. Then knowing your allowable calorie total for the meal, decide how much to eat – and take the remainder home. If fresh fruit is not an option, pass on dessert and have the evening snack specified for that day on this diet.

In a restaurant, most nutritionists recommend you eat the low-calorie items on your plate first. Start with the salad, soup and veggies. By the time you get to the legumes and starches you will hopefully be full enough to be content with smaller portions of the higher-calorie choices.

Incidentally, if you live in a small town with no vegetarian restaurant, to stay on this diet, have a frozen vegetarian entree. And try to abide by the allowable calorie total.

Finally, some dieticians advise their dieting clients not to eat out. That's right. They believe eating at home is safer. But our thought is you have to eat out eventually so why not learn how while your resolve is high?

Diet Tip of the Day: To determine your frame size, circle your wrist with your thumb and third finger. If the tips of your fingers overlap, you have a small frame. If they just touch you are medium, and if they don't touch you have a large frame.

Day 36 - Recipe

Grilled Tilapia

Tilapia is a mild, white fish that inhabits fresh water. This fish has very low levels of mercury because it's fast-growing, short-lived, and mostly eats a vegetarian diet. According to the Monterey Bay Aquarium, choose tilapia farmed in the U.S., in environmentally friendly systems. "Avoid" farmed tilapia from China and Taiwan, where pollution and weak management are a problem.

    4 Tilapia filets (about 6 ounces each)

Marinade: ¾ cup olive oil, ½ lemon, juiced, 1 tablespoons oregano, ½ teaspoon black pepper, ¼ cup red wine vinegar, ½ cup finely chopped parsley, 2 cloves garlic, minced and 2 dashes Tabasco (optional).

Combine all ingredients (except filets) in a large re-sealable plastic bag and shake well. Then place fish filets in the marinade for 30 minutes. Remove fillets from marinade and cook on hot grill for approximately 2 to 3 minutes per side.

Serves 4. About 300 Calories per serving (fish only)

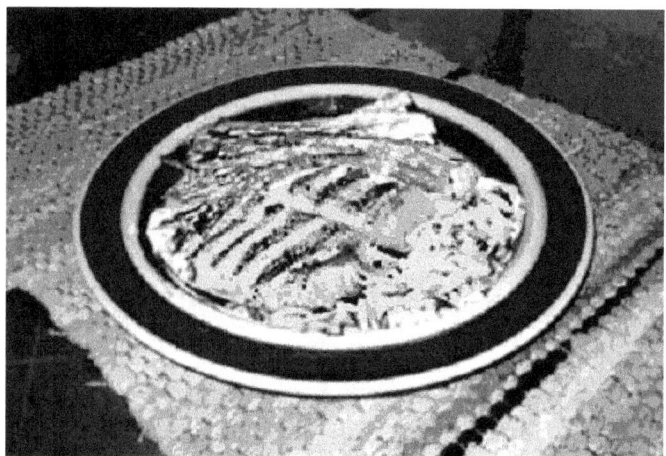

Photo shows two fish filets. Actual serving size is one filet.

Diet Tip of the Day: One serving of asparagus can provide you with 66% of your daily folate needs. Folate is a B-vitamin which is involved with cellular division, and therefore aids the development of a baby's nervous system.

Day 37 - Recipe

Bulgur & Veggies

¾ cups bulgur, dry
1 bunch Kale (about 1 lb)
2 medium sweet potatoes, cut in
8 medium button mushrooms
2 tablespoons olive oil, divided

1. Cook bulgur according to package directions.
2. Clean and quarter mushrooms. Over medium heat sauté mushrooms in olive oil until they turn reddish brown with golden spots, about 10 minutes.
3. Cut sweet potatoes into bite-size pieces. Place in baking pan and coat potatoes lightly with olive oil. Roast in oven set at 375°F for about 25 minutes, or until done.
4. Wash kale and remove kale stems. Chop and then steam until tender.

Serves 4. About 270 Calories per serving

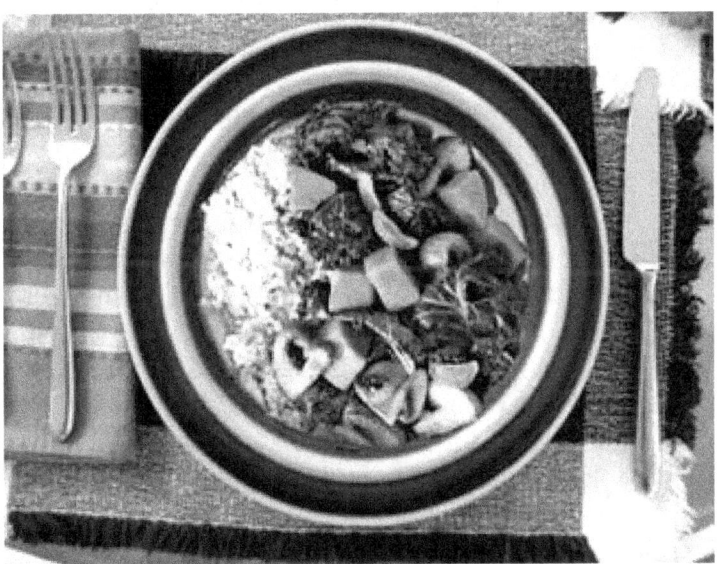

Diet Tip of the Day: According to a study published in the Journal of Food Chemistry, broccoli, spinach, kale, Brussels sprouts and other dark green vegetables have the highest cancer-fighting potential found in produce.

Day 38 - Recipe

Risotto Primavera

    5 cups low-sodium vegetable broth
    3 tablespoons olive oil, divided
    3 tablespoons butter, divided
    ½ large yellow onion, finely diced
    3 carrots, finely diced
    1 cup cauliflower and broccoli pieces
    1 yellow squash, diced
    1½ cups Arborio rice
    1½ cups white wine
    4 green onions, thinly sliced
    ½ cup frozen peas
    4 ounces goat cheese
    ½ cup grated Parmesan cheese

1. Pour vegetable broth into a small saucepan. Heat to a simmer.
2. In large Dutch oven, heat 2 tablespoons olive oil and 2 tablespoons butter. Add diced onions and carrots. Stir and cook for about 1 minute. Add cauliflower and cook for another minute. Add broccoli and cook for 30 seconds. Then add squash and cook for 30 seconds. Sprinkle in salt and stir. Remove from Dutch oven and put on a plate. Set aside.
3. Add 1 tablespoon olive oil and 1 tablespoon butter to the Dutch oven. Over medium-low heat, add rice and stir, cooking for 1 minute. Add half the wine and 1½ teaspoons kosher salt. Stir and cook until liquid is absorbed. Over the next 30 to 45 minutes, add 1 cup of simmering vegetable broth from the small saucepan at a time, stirring and cooking until each addition of broth has been absorbed. Add other half cup of wine and cook until absorbed. Add green onions and peas, stirring to combine. Taste to make sure rice is the right texture.
4. Once rice is cooked, remove from heat. Stir in goat cheese, Parmesan cheese, and vegetables until all goat cheese is combined. Serve on a plate with a sprig of dill.
Serves 8. About 365 Calories per serving

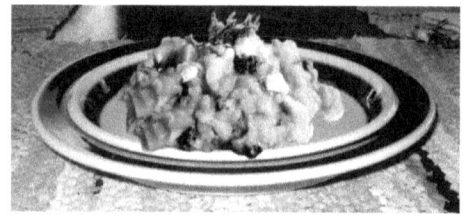

Day 39 - Recipe

Tofu Steak with Veggies

⅓ cup white miso (soybean paste)
⅓ cup mirin (sweet rice wine)
⅓ cup rice vinegar
1 tablespoon finely grated peeled fresh ginger
½ cup chopped dry-roasted peanuts, divided
5 tablespoons sesame oil, divided
2 (14-ounce) packages water-packed firm tofu, drained
8 cups salad greens

1. Combine white miso, mirin, ¼ cup peanuts, and 3 tablespoons oil in a small bowl; stir with a whisk.
2. Cut each tofu block crosswise into 8 (½-inch-thick) slices. Arrange tofu on several layers of paper towels. Top with several more layers of paper towels; top with a cast-iron skillet or other heavy pan. Let stand 30 minutes. Remove tofu from paper towels.
3. Heat 1 tablespoon oil in a large nonstick skillet over medium-high heat. Add 4 tofu slices to pan; sauté 4 minutes on each side or until crisp and golden. Remove from pan, and drain tofu on paper towels. Repeat procedure with remaining 1 tablespoon oil and remaining 4 tofu slices.
4. Place 1 cup greens on each of 8 plates. Top each serving with 2 tofu slices, 3 tablespoons miso mixture, and 1½ teaspoons chopped peanuts.

Serves 8: About 275 Calories per serving.

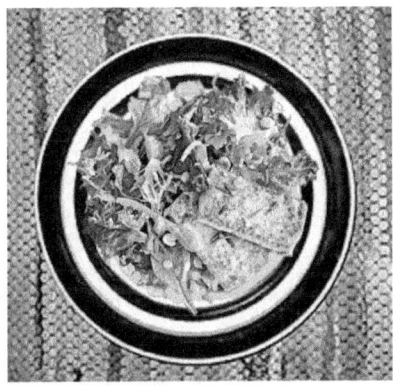

Diet Tip of the Day: Steaming in a microwave oven is one of the best ways to cook veggies so they retain nutrients. Another advantage is the cooking adds no fat or sodium.

Day 40 - Recipe

Fish Dinner - Out

No recipe today. No cooking today. Have a fish dinner at your favorite restaurant, but make sure you choose a restaurant where you have a good chance to achieve your calorie goal. For today, your **goal for dinner is a maximum of 595 Calories**. This includes appetizer, soup, main course and dessert.

Tips for Eating Fish Out: The following is almost an exact repeat of the advice given eating out on previous days. First, order simple, such as broiled fish with steamed vegetables and brown rice. Tell the waiter you want no sauce, no gravy, nothing added. Then, knowing your calorie objective, and that fish is about 50 Calories per ounce, most steamed vegetable servings average approximately 50 Calories per cup, and rice is about 100 Calories per ½ cup, decide how much to eat – and take the remainder home. If fresh fruit is not an option, pass on dessert and have the evening snack specified for that day in the diet.

In a restaurant, some nutritionists recommend you eat the low-calorie items on your plate first. Start with the salad, soup and veggies. By the time you get to the fish and starches you will hopefully be full enough to be content with smaller portions of the higher-calorie choices.

Diet Tip of the Day: The average egg has only 210 mg of cholesterol (found in the yoke), contains 80 calories, many vitamins many minerals. If you're healthy and your LDL blood cholesterol level is low, many experts feel you can safely eat one egg per day.

Day 41 - Recipe

Pasta e Fagioli

This is a variation of a nutritious peasant dish served all over Italy.

- 14.5-oz can whole tomatoes with juice, crushed
- 14.5-oz can cannellini beans, drained
- 1 cup of any tube-shaped pasta
- 2 tablespoon olive oil
- 1 medium onion, diced
- 2 cloves garlic, minced
- 1 stalk celery, finely chopped
- 3 cups chicken stock
- 2 cups fresh baby spinach or escarole
- 1 tsp dried basil
- ½ teaspoon dried oregano
- 2 Tbsp fresh parsley, chopped

Heat olive oil, onion and celery in large saucepan over medium heat. Sauté until onions are golden brown. Add garlic and stir constantly for one minute. Pour in tomatoes and their juices and bring to a boil. Add beans and chicken stock and return to a boil. Stir in spinach (or escarole) and seasonings. Simmer for about 5 minutes. Add pasta and cook about 15 minutes or until pasta is tender but firm. If needed, thin soup with hot water. Ladle into soup bowls. Garnish with grated Parmesan cheese. Salt and pepper to taste.

Serves 4. About 300 Calories per serving.

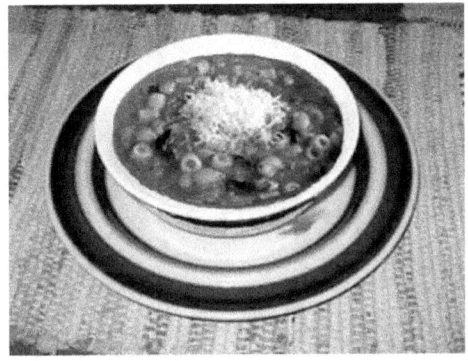

Diet Tip of the Day: Pasta alone is an incomplete protein. But when combined with beans, a complete protein results – that is a protein that contains all eight essential amino acids. The dish is every bit as nutritious as meat, fish or poultry.

Day 42 - Recipe

Dawn's Blueberry Muffins

Wholesome whole-wheat blueberry muffins just like grandma used to make. Serve them at breakfast, or as a nutritious dessert, or a wonderful snack. (Make a dozen. Have one today and store remainder in your freezer until they are called for again later in the diet.)

   4 ounces bran flakes
   ¼ cup sugar
   1¼ cups whole wheat flour
   1 teaspoon baking soda
   ¼ teaspoon baking powder
   ¼ teaspoon salt
   ½ cup blueberries (fresh or frozen)
   1 egg, beaten
   1 cup buttermilk
   ¼ cup vegetable oil

Preheat oven to 400 °F. Coat muffin tins with nonstick cooking spray. In a bowl combine dry ingredients. In another bowl combine wet ingredients and mix thoroughly. Add wet ingredients to dry ingredients and mix until just blended. Do not over mix. Gently fold in blueberries. Spoon batter into muffin tins until two-thirds full. Bake 15 minutes or until muffin tops are golden brown.

Yield is 12 Muffins, 145 Calories each

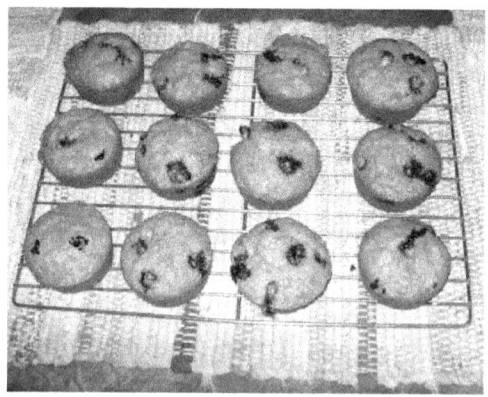

Diet Tip of the Day: **Acquire a good low-calorie cookbook**. Be sure the recipes cover breakfast, lunch and dinner, and all the recipes contain nutritional information, especially the calories per serving.

Day 43 - Recipe

Halibut & Corn

   1 pound halibut filet, divided into 4 portions
   2 teaspoons olive oil, divided
   1 package store-bought tomato-pineapple salsa
   4 whole beets

1. Pat halibut filets dry and dust lightly with all-purpose flour. Salt and pepper to taste.
2. In large skillet over medium heat, sauté halibut in 1 teaspoon olive oil with squeeze of lemon for 2 minutes on each side.
3. Plate halibut with 2 tablespoons salsa.
4. Roast whole beets in their skin for about 45 minutes. Peel and cut into cubes. Toss in remaining olive oil.

Serves 4. About 175 Calories per serving (salad and corn not included).

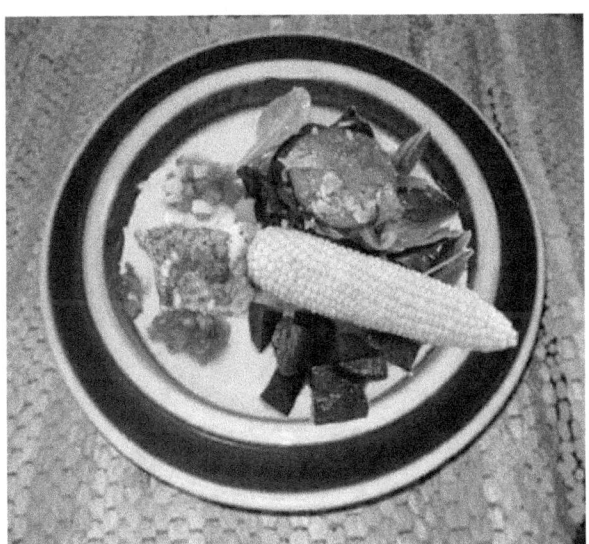

Diet Tip of the Day: Remember your stomach is about the size of your fist. So it doesn't take much food to fill it comfortably.

Day 44 - Recipe

<u>Baked Haddock</u>

4   4-oz haddock fillets (or salmon fillets)
½   cup white wine
½   cup non-fat yogurt mixed with ¼ cup pureed roasted red pepper
½   pound green beans
¾   pint cherry tomatoes (about 20)
1   tablespoon olive oil
¾   cup bulgur, prepared per package directions

Lightly dust fillets with flour. Dip in beaten egg white and then in Panko bread crumbs. Brown fillets in non-stick pan. Place fillets skin side down in baking dish coated with non-stick spray. Add white wine and cook in oven preheated to 350 °F for about 15 minutes. Spoon pan juices over fillets. Salt and pepper to taste.

Place green beans in skillet. Add ¼-inch of water and cook over medium heat until water boils off. Add cherry tomatoes and olive oil. Stir well and sauté for a few minutes. Season with fresh rosemary and oregano. Salt and pepper to taste.

Plate haddock fillet and spoon over yogurt-red pepper sauce. Garnish with fresh parsley. Add green beans & tomato mix and the bulgur. Serve hot.

<u>Serves 4</u>. One plate consisting of one haddock fillet (215 Calories) with green beans & tomato mix (65 Calories) and bulgur (140 Calories) totals 420 Calories.

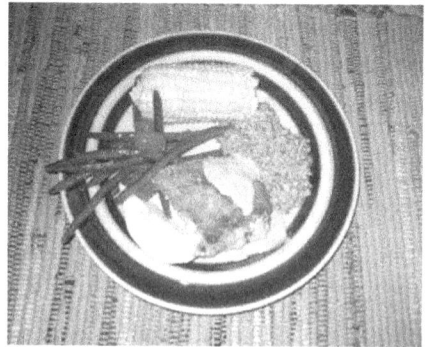

Note that corn-on-the-cob is only for the 1,800 Calorie diet.

<u>Diet Tip of the Day:</u> It's much easier to stay with an exercise program when it's done in tandem. So enlist a friend to be your exercise buddy.

Day 45 - Recipe

Quinoa with Veggies Salad

1 cup water
½ cup uncooked quinoa
¾ cup fresh parsley leaves
½ cup thinly sliced celery
½ cup thinly sliced green onions
½ cup finely chopped dried apricots
3 tablespoons fresh lemon juice
1 tablespoon olive oil
1 tablespoon honey
¼ teaspoon salt
¼ teaspoon black pepper
¼ cup unsalted pumpkin seed kernels, toasted

1. Bring water and quinoa to a boil in a medium saucepan. Cover, reduce heat, and simmer 20 minutes or until liquid is absorbed.
2. Spoon into a bowl and fluff with a fork. Add parsley, celery, onions, and apricots.
3. Whisk lemon juice, olive oil, honey, salt, and black pepper. Add to quinoa mixture, and toss well. Top with pumpkin seeds. Serve at room temperature.

Serves 4. 240 Cal per serving

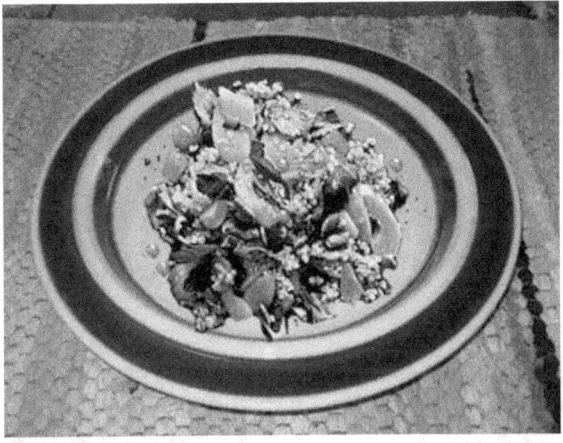

Diet Tip of the Day: Inevitably, you're going to be faced with a stressful situation. Instead of turning to food for comfort, be prepared with some non-food tactics that work for you, such as listening to music, reading, writing in a journal, or meditating.

Day 46 - Recipe

Poached Cod in Tomato Broth

- 2 cups dry white wine
- 1 cup clam juice
- 2 cans (14.5-ounce) diced tomatoes, drained
- 1 small onion, diced
- 1 garlic clove, minced
- ½ tsp dried parsley, or sprigs of fresh parsley
- 1 bay leaf
- 12 black olives, pitted and halved
- 4 cod fish fillets (about 6 ounces each)

Note that sole, flounder, halibut or haddock may be substituted for cod.

Use a pan large enough to hold the fish in a single layer. Place all the ingredients except the fish in the pan. Over high heat, bring poaching liquid to a boil (pan uncovered). Reduce heat and simmer the liquid another 6 minutes.

Carefully place the fish filets in the liquid. Cover the pan and reduce heat until liquid is just simmering. Poach until fish are completely opaque and tender – about 8 minutes. Plate fish and ladle broth over fish.

<u>Serves 4</u>. 275 Calories per serving.

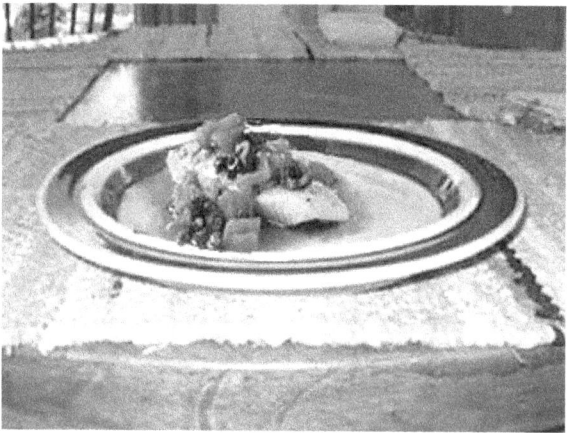

<u>Diet Tip of the Day:</u> A **good reducing diet must help you remain healthy** while you are losing weight.

Day 47 - Recipe

Healthy Pasta Salad

½ pound fusilli pasta, cooked until tender but firm
2 broccoli crowns, chopped
¼ pint cherry tomatoes (about 8), halved
½ cup black olives, halved
½ cup garbanzo beans (chick peas)
½ cup fresh "light" mozzarella, chopped
1 tablespoon basil
1 tablespoon rosemary
2 teaspoons garlic powder
¼ cup of a **recommended dressing** (see page 12)

Combine dry ingredients in a medium-size bowl. Stir in salad dressing.
Mix thoroughly. Salt and black pepper to taste.

Serves 4. 370 Calories per serving.

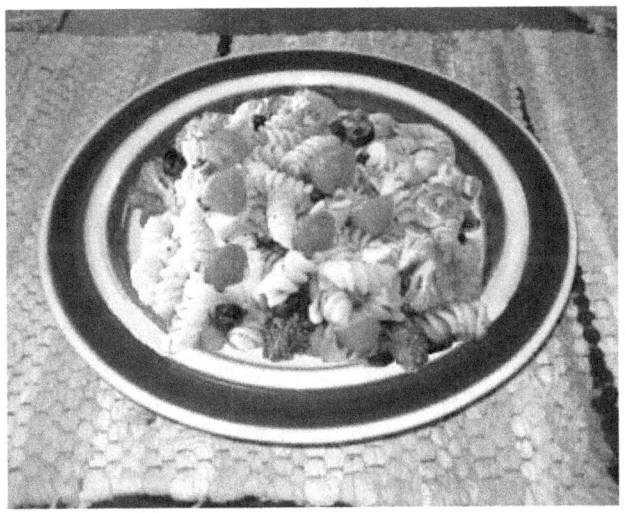

Diet Tip of the Day: Ask yourself: **"Why am I overweight?"** Do you
eat too much of everything? Too much dessert? Drink too much beer? Is
your only exercise walking from the TV to the refrigerator? Determine the
why and then focus on one or two of your problem areas. Sometimes it's
that simple.

Day 48 - Recipe

<u>Vegetarian Dinner - Out</u>

No recipe today. No cooking today. Have dinner at your favorite vegetarian restaurant, but make sure you choose a restaurant where you have a fighting chance to achieve your calorie goal. For your vegetarian dinner out, your maximum allowable calories (including appetizer, soup, main course and dessert) are as follows:

- For the **1,200 Calorie Diet**: 530 Calories
- For the **1,500 Calorie Diet**: 630 Calories

Tips for Eating Vegetarian Out: First, order simple such as tofu stir fried with vegetables, and brown rice. Tell the waiter you want little to no added sauce or gravy. Estimate the calories in the meal: tofu is about 75 Calories per ounce, most vegetable servings average approximately 50 Calories per cup, rice is about 100 Calories per ½ cup, and add about 150 Calories for the oil used in the stir fry. Then knowing your allowable calorie total for the meal, decide how much to eat – and take the remainder home. If fresh fruit is not an option, pass on dessert and have the evening snack specified for that day on this diet.

In a restaurant, most nutritionists recommend you eat the low-calorie items on your plate first. Start with the salad, soup and veggies. By the time you get to the legumes and starches you will hopefully be full enough to be content with smaller portions of the higher-calorie choices.

Incidentally, if you live in a small town with no vegetarian restaurant, to stay on this diet, have a frozen vegetarian entree. And try to abide by the allowable calorie total.

Finally, some dieticians advise their dieting clients not to eat out. That's right. They believe eating at home is safer. But our thought is you have to eat out eventually so why not learn how while your resolve is high?

<u>Diet Tip of the Day:</u> Inevitably, everyone on a diet hits a frustrating **weight-loss plateau**. Two ways to bust through the plateau are: first to reduce your calorie intake and second to step up your exercise intensity.

Day 49 - Recipe

Frozen Pasta Dinner

No recipe today. No cooking today. It's your day off! Some reasonably good frozen pasta dinners are:

- Lean Cuisine Angel Hair Pomodoro (220 Cal)
- Lean Cuisine Cheese Ravioli (250 Cal)
- Healthy Choice Portobella Spinach Parmesan (230 Cal)
- Healthy Choice Portobella Marsala Pasta (230 Cal)
- Amy's Light & Lean Spagehetti Italiano (240 Cal)

If you choose any of the above entrees, you will not use all of the **300 Calories allocated for this meal**. In this case, use the excess 100 or so calories anyway you wish. Splurge on extra dessert or save the calories for another day!

Please read the important **Frozen-Food Safety Warning** in **Appendix C** on page 209.

Diet Tip of the Day: Experts agree that whether you are trying to lose weight or just maintain your weight, **it's calories that count**. It doesn't matter what foods the calories are from. To lose weight you must eat fewer calories than you burn. Calories count! Not carbs, not Weight Watchers points. Calories – period!

Day 50 - Recipe

Pan-Fried Sole

   4   sole fillets (6-ounces each), skinned
   1   tablespoon olive oil

Salsa Ingredients:

   1 pint cherry tomatoes, quartered
   ¾ cup cucumber, finely chopped
   ⅓ cup yellow bell pepper, finely chopped
   3 tablespoons fresh basil, chopped
   2 tablespoons capers
   1½ tablespoons shallots, finely chopped
   1 tablespoon balsamic vinegar
   2 teaspoons lemon rind, grated

Combine salsa ingredients in a bowl and stir in ½ teaspoon salt and ⅛ teaspoon black pepper. Mix thoroughly.

Heat olive oil in a large nonstick skillet over medium-high heat. Season sole fillets with
½ teaspoon salt and ⅛ teaspoon black pepper. Add fish to pan; cook about 1½ minutes on each side or until fish flakes easily when tested with a fork. Spoon salsa over fish and serve immediately.

<u>Serves 4</u>. 325 Calories per serving

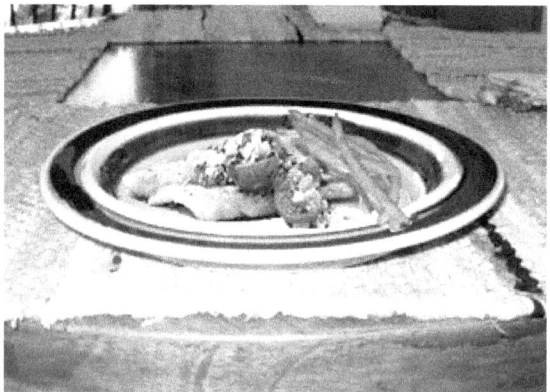

<u>Diet Tip of the Day:</u> If you are overweight start on a weight loss diet now because it will only become **more difficult to lose weight as you get older**.

Day 51 - Recipe

Beans & Greens Salad (Repeated)

⅓ cup chopped oregano
⅓ cup chopped parsley
3 cloves garlic, chopped
1 lemon, juiced

Prepare dressing by combining above ingredients and stirring in ¼ cup extra-virgin olive oil. Salt and pepper to taste.
½ pound mesclun mix
¼ pound green beans
19-ounce can garbanzo beans (chickpeas)
Arrange mesclun mix, garbanzo beans and green beans on a large platter. Drizzle dressing over beans and greens.

<u>Serves 4</u>. Approximately 260 Calories per serving.

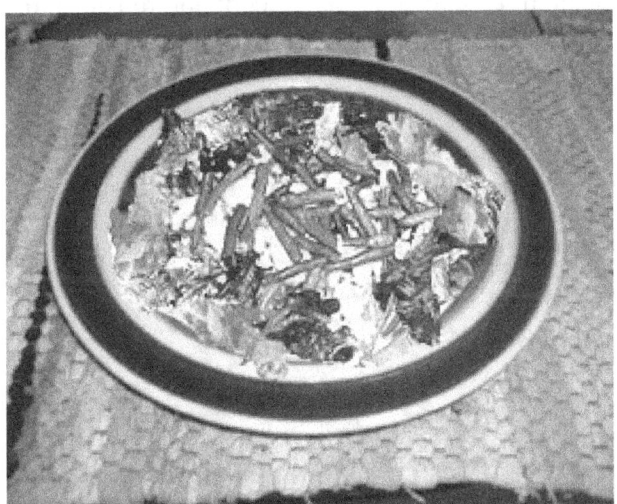

<u>Diet Tip of the Day:</u> **Fat-free isn't always your best bet**. Low fat doesn't necessarily mean low calorie! Most often sugar is substituted for fat and the calorie total remains the same or even higher. Instead, look for low-calorie or reduced-calorie foods.

Day 52 - Recipe

Bay Scallops & Snow Peas

For Pesceterians that do not eat scallops, please skip this meal.

> 1 tablespoon olive oil
> 1 large shallot, diced
> 5 ounces button mushrooms, chopped coarsely
> 3 ounces snow peas, halved
> ¼ teaspoon ground lemon pepper
> 1 tablespoon rice vinegar
> ⅛ teaspoon (or less) red pepper flakes
> ½ pound bay scallops
> ¼ teaspoon thyme
> ¼ teaspoon tarragon

1. Heat olive oil in a skillet over medium heat. Add shallot and mushrooms. Sauté until shallot is translucent and mushrooms are cooked.
2. Stir in snow peas and remaining ingredients except scallops, thyme and tarragon. Cook for about 2 minutes.
3. Add scallops, stirring often, and cook another 3 minutes, or until scallops are white, not translucent, on all sides.
4. Stir in thyme and tarragon and cook for another thirty seconds.
5. Plate and serve.

Serves 2. 240 Calories per serving.

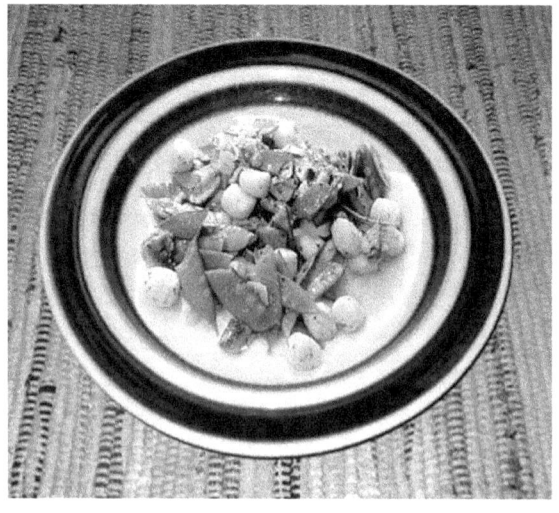

Day 53 - Recipe

Tofu, Bok Choy & Mushroom Stir Fry

2 (14-ounce) packages water-packed firm tofu, drained
2 tablespoons sesame oil
3 cloves minced garlic
½ cup sliced shiitake mushrooms
½ cup sliced button mushrooms
2 teaspoons canola oil
1 tablespoon soy sauce
1 bok choy, chopped (or 2 to 3 baby bok choy)
6 scallions (green onions), sliced
¼ cup vegetable broth
2 teaspoons fresh ginger, grated
2 teaspoons sesame oil

1) Go to page 207 for instruction re preparation of tofu steaks. (Cut each tofu block crosswise into 8 (½-inch-thick) slices.)
2) Sauté garlic and mushrooms in canola oil for 3 to 5 minutes. Add in soy sauce, bok choy and scallions, and cook for about 3 more minutes.
3) Reduce heat to medium low and add vegetable broth and ginger. Simmer for another 3 to 5 minutes.
4) Stir in the sesame oil and remove from heat.
5) Serve bok choy and mushroom stir-fry with 2 tofu steaks over brown rice.

Serves 4. About 330 Calories per serving (including tofu but not the rice).

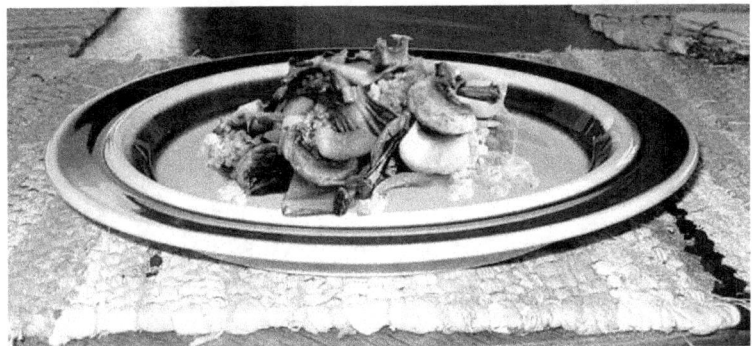

Tofu steaks not shown in photo.

Diet Tip of the Day: Bear in mind, that knowledge and the discipline to **workout regularly** are far more important than fancy equipment.

Day 54 - Recipe

<u>Vegetables with Couscous</u>

    1 10-ounce box couscous
    1 red bell pepper, cut into strips
    1 yellow bell pepper, cut into strips
    1 small yellow squash, sliced
    1 small zucchini, sliced
    1 teaspoon salt
    ¾ teaspoon black pepper
    ¾ teaspoon minced garlic
    ¾ teaspoon Italian seasoning
    2 tablespoon olive oil
    3 tablespoon balsamic vinegar
    5 ounces feta cheese

1. Pre-heat oven to 425 °F.
2. Prepare couscous according to package directions.
3. In a small bowl, whisk together marinade of salt, pepper, garlic, Italian seasoning, olive oil and balsamic vinegar and toss with pepper strips, sliced squash and zucchini.
4. Spread vegetables evenly in sheet pan and roast for 10 to 12 minutes or until vegetables are crisp-tender. Reserve left over marinade.
5. Allow vegetables to cool slightly, then toss with remaining marinade, couscous and feta cheese.

<u>Serves 6</u>. About 310 Calories per serving

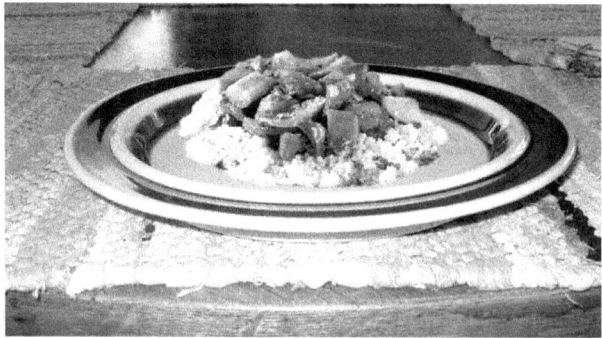

<u>Diet Tip of the Day</u>: To make sure you stay on track, **weigh in once a week**. There may be times when you might not see a weight loss, often because lost fat is temporarily replaced by water. This condition will gradually be corrected as you continue dieting.

Day 55 - Recipe

Hearty Vegetable Soup

2 15-oz cans white kidney beans, drained
1 tablespoon olive oil
½ large yellow onion, chopped
2 garlic cloves, minced
1 cup chopped fresh tomatoes
2 celery stalks, cut into ½-inch pieces
1½ carrots, cut into ½-inch pieces
5 cups vegetable stock
1 medium potato, cut into ½-inch pieces
¼ cup chopped fresh basil
¼ head of red cabbage, cut into ½-inch pieces
2 zucchini or summer squash, cut into ½-inch pieces

Heat olive oil in a large pot over medium heat. Add onion and garlic.
Sauté 5 minutes. Add green cabbage, tomatoes, celery, and carrots. Sauté
an additional 10 minutes. Add beans, 5 cups of vegetable stock, potatoes,
and basil. Bring to a boil. Reduce heat, cover and simmer for one hour.
Add red cabbage, zucchini and salt . Cover and simmer until vegetables are
tender, about 20 minutes longer. Stir in about ¼ cup Parmesan cheese and
sprinkle a dash of Tabasco hot sauce if you want a little zip.

Serves 4. 360 Calories per serving

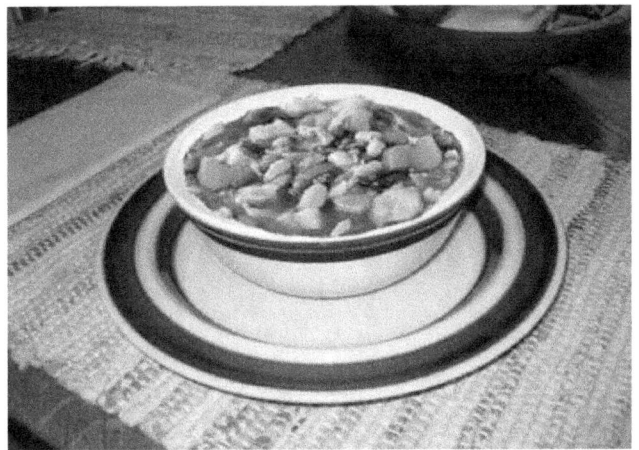

Diet Tip of the Day: Water and fiber contain no calories – that is **zero
Calories** per ounce.

Day 56 - Recipe

Frozen Tofu-based Dinner

No recipe today. No cooking today. It's your day off! Some reasonably good frozen tofu-based dinners are:

- Amy's Tofu Scramble (320 Cal)
- Amy's Thai Stir Fry (310 Cal)
- Amy's Teriyaki Bowl (290 Cal)
- Amy's Brown Rice & Vegetables Bowl (260 Cal)

That's it. At this writing, there are just not that many frozen Tofu-based dinners for sale at supermarkets, although there could be new entrees introduced after this book "went to press." If you choose any of the above entrees, you will not use all of the **340 Calories allocated for this meal**. In this case, use the excess 100 or so calories anyway you wish. Splurge on extra dessert or save the calories for another day!

Please read the important **Frozen-Food Safety Warning** in **Appendix C** on page 209.

Diet Tip of the Day: To prevent or delay the onset of type II diabetes, experts urge the overweight to lose weight and work out regularly. Weight loss helps your body use insulin more efficiently, and exercise helps metabolize excess circulating blood glucose.

Day 57 - Recipe

Salmon with Mango Salsa

  4 salmon fillets (about 5 ounces each)
1½ pounds baby new potatoes, halved
  1 mango, ripe
  3 green onions, finely chopped
  3 tablespoons chopped fresh cilantro
  2 tablespoons lemon juice
  2 teaspoons extra-virgin olive oil
  4 cups watercress

Remove any tiny bones from salmon. Press crushed peppercorns into flesh side of salmon. Set aside. Place halved potatoes into saucepan. Cover with water and bring to a boil. Reduce the heat and simmer until tender, about 10-12 minutes and drain.

Prepare salsa: Peel and seed the mango. Dice the mango flesh and put into a large bowl. Mix in green onions, cilantro, lemon juice, olive oil, and an optional dash of Tabasco.

Heat a grill pan coated with nonstick cooking spray over medium-high heat. Place salmon fillets in pan, skin-side down. Cook for 4 minutes. Turn fish over and cook until done, about another 4 minutes. Arrange watercress and new potatoes on serving plates. Place salmon on top and spoon over mango salsa.

Serves 4. 460 Calories per serving

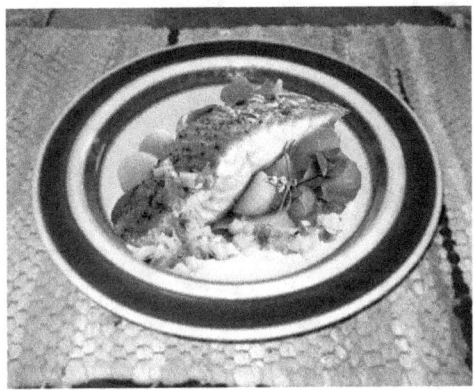

Diet Tip of the Day: All **foods are a combination of water, carbohydrate, protein, fat and fiber**. Knowing this can lead to a better understanding of why a food has a particular caloric value.

Day 58 - Recipe
Tofu & Broccoli in Garlic Sauce

1 medium onion, diced
4 cloves garlic, minced
3 tablespoon olive oil
2 cups broccoli, chopped
1 (14-ounce) package water-packed firm tofu, drained
1½ teaspoons ginger powder
¼ teaspoon cayenne pepper
3 tablespoon corn starch
¼ cup soy sauce
1 cup water

1. See page 207 for Tofu preparation instructions. (Cut tofu into 1-inch cubes.)
2. In a large skillet, over medium heat, sauté onions and garlic in olive oil until onions turn clear, about 3-5 minutes.
3. Add the tofu, ginger, cayenne and broccoli to the pan and continue to cook until broccoli is done, another 6-8 minutes.
4. In a separate small bowl, mix together the corn starch, soy sauce and water. Then add this mixture to the broccoli and tofu. Cook until sauce thickens, then remove from heat.
5. Serve over brown rice.

Serves 4. About 320 Calories per serving (not including rice).

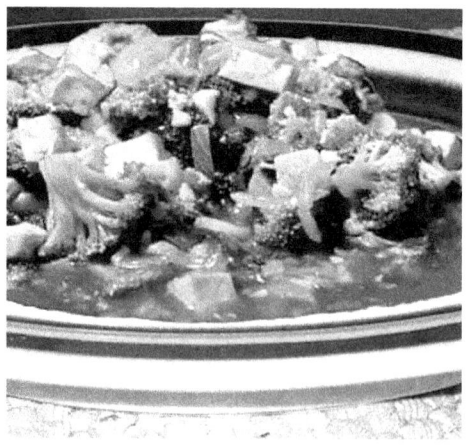

Diet Tip of the Day: Tofu typically contains about 1¼ Calories per gram - depending on how it is prepared (baked, fried, etc.)

Day 59 - Recipe

Pasta-Based Dinner - Out

No recipe today. No cooking today. Have a pasta dinner at your favorite Italian restaurant, but make sure you choose a restaurant where you have a reasonable chance to achieve your calorie goal. For today, **your goal for dinner is a maximum of 640 Calories**. This includes any appetizer, soup, main course and any dessert.

Tips for Eating Pasta: Americans adore Italian food. But you can consume a lot of calories in an Italian restaurant – if you order carelessly. For example a typical portion of Fried calamari with garlic bread totals more than 1,100 Calories!

First rule, order simple. Look for pasta in a marinara sauce and a salad with dressing on the side. Then, knowing your 640 Calorie objective, and that most pastas are about 50 Calories per ounce, and marinara tomato sauce averages about 70 Calories per half cup, decide how much of the meal you can eat – and take the remainder home. To stay within your maximum allowable calorie total, you should pass on dessert and have the evening snack specified for that day in the diet.

Diet Tip of the Day: A handful of studies suggest that chewing gum may help reduce your craving for sweet snacks, and cut your caloric intake by about 50 per day. Another study actually showed that gum chewers experienced a small increase in their daily energy expenditure. And gum adds hardly any calories to your diet. Regular gum has about 10 calories and sugar-free varieties about five calories per stick.

Day 60 - Recipe

Cashew Tofu Stir Fry

3 cloves garlic, minced
1 teaspoon fresh ginger, minced
2 tablespoons peanut oil
8 ounces extra-firm tofu, pressed
¾ cup mushrooms, sliced
1 4-ounce can bamboo shoots, drained & sliced thin
2 stalks celery, sliced
1 large green bell pepper, chopped
⅓ cup vegetable broth
2 tablespoons soy sauce
1 tablespoon cornstarch mixed with 3 tablespoons water
½ cup cashews
3 green onions, chopped

1. For tofu draining and preparation tips see page 207. (Cut tofu into 1-inch cubes.)
2. In a large skillet or wok, heat oil and add garlic and ginger for about 2 minutes. Then add the tofu, carefully stirring to mix up the ginger and garlic. Cook for 3 to 4 minutes, or until tofu is lightly golden.
3. Add bell pepper and celery, and cook, stirring for about a minute. Then add mushrooms and bamboo shoots.
4. Add vegetable broth and soy sauce. Allow to simmer for another minute or two, until vegetables are tender but not yet done.
5. Stir in water-cornstarch mixture, heat until thickened and vegetables are done. Then stir in cashews and green onions, to combine well. Serve over steamed white rice.

Serves 4. About 275 Calories per serving (not including rice).

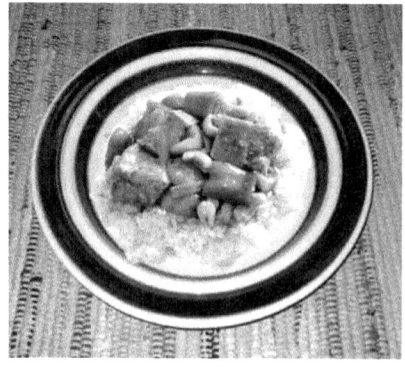

Day 61 - Recipe

Shells with Cheese & Walnuts

½ cup walnuts 325
2 cloves garlic 10
1 tablespoon olive 115
1 box medium whole-wheat shells 1600
1 pound frozen peas 350
6 ounces goat cheese 615

1) Heat covered 6-quart pot of water to boiling on high. Add 2 teaspoons salt.
2) In an 8- to 10-inch skillet, combine walnuts, garlic, and oil. Cook on medium until golden and fragrant, stirring occasionally. Stir in 1/8 teaspoon each salt and freshly ground black pepper.
3) Add pasta to boiling water in pot. Cook 1 minute less than minimum time that label directs, stirring occasionally. Add peas; cook 1 minute longer. Reserve 1 cup pasta cooking water. Drain pasta and peas; return to pot.
4) Add goat cheese, 1/2 cup cooking water, 1/4 teaspoon salt, and 1/2 teaspoon freshly ground black pepper. If mixture is dry, toss with additional cooking water.
5) To serve, top with garlic-and-walnut mixture.

Serves 4. 490 Calories per serving

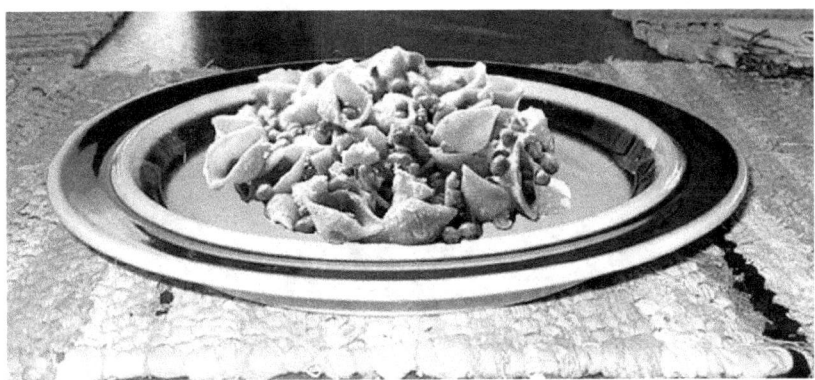

Diet Tip of the Day: If your caloric intake on a weight-loss diet is constant, your **rate of weight loss will decrease with time**. So if you want to lose weight at a constant rate over time, you must eat slightly less (or exercise harder) as you lose weight.

Day 62 - Recipe

Curried Eggplant & Tomato

1 cup white basmati rice
1 tablespoon olive oil
1 onion, chopped
2 pints cherry tomatoes, halved
1 eggplant (about 1 pound), cut into ½-inch pieces
1 15.5-ounce can chickpeas, rinsed
1½ teaspoons curry powder
½ cup fresh basil

1) In medium saucepan with a tight-fitting lid, combine rice, 1½ cups water, and ½ teaspoon salt and bring to a boil. Stir rice once, cover, and reduce heat to low. Simmer for about 18 minutes. Remove from heat and let stand, covered, for 5 minutes.
2) Meanwhile, cook oil in saucepan over medium-high heat. Add onion and cook, stirring occasionally, until softened, 4 to 6 minutes.
3) Stir in tomatoes, eggplant, curry powder, 1 teaspoon salt, and ¼ teaspoon black pepper. Cook, stirring, until fragrant, about 2 minutes.
4) Add 2 cups water and bring to a boil. Reduce heat and simmer, partially covered, until eggplant is tender, about 12 to 15 minutes. Stir in chickpeas and cook until heated through, about 3 minutes.
5) Remove vegetables from heat and stir in basil. Fluff rice with a fork. Serve vegetables over steamed white rice.

Serves 4. About 325 Calories per serving (including rice).

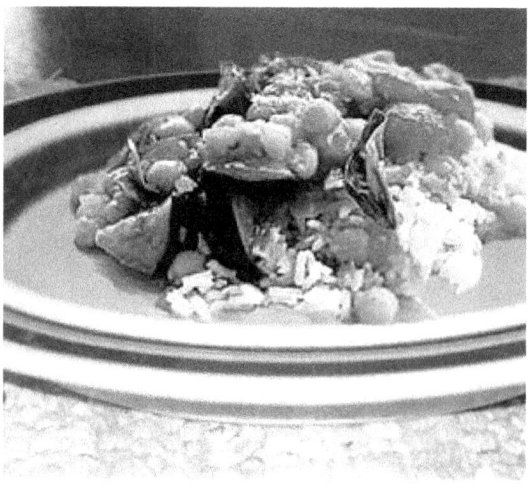

Day 63 - Recipe

Indian Shahi Paneer

 2 tablespoons cooking oil
 1 large onion, thinly sliced
 4 cloves garlic, minced
 1 teaspoon ground cumin
 1 teaspoon ground coriander
 ½ teaspoon ground turmeric
 ½ teaspoon red chili powder
 4 tomatoes, pureed
 ½ pound paneer, cubed
 1 teaspoon sugar
 ¼ cup cream
 2 tablespoons chopped fresh cilantro

1) Cook oil in a large skillet over medium heat. Add onion and garlic in the hot oil until the onions are soft and golden brown, about 5 minutes. Sprinkle in cumin, coriander, turmeric, and chili powder over onion and garlic. Continue cooking until seasonings are fragrant, about 30 seconds.
2) Pour pureed tomatoes into skillet. Cook until excess liquid evaporates and oil separates, 3 to 5 minutes. Add paneer, ¼ cup water, sugar, and salt to mixture. Stir gently so paneer does not break apart. Cook until paneer begins to absorb some of liquid, about 10 minutes.
3) Stir cream into mixture and simmer another 5 minutes. Salt to taste. Serve with garnish of cilantro over steamed white rice.
Serves 4. About 230 Calories per serving.

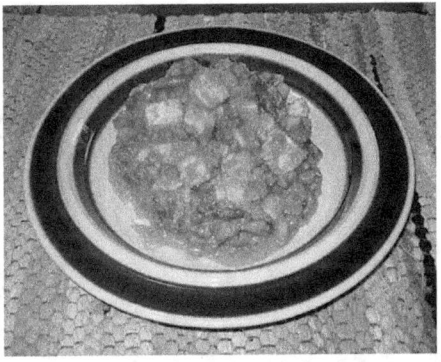

Diet Tip of the Day: **Working out at home** has some significant advantages. It takes less time because you don't have to drive back and forth to a fitness facility; and working out at home is less expensive.

Day 64 - Recipe

Grilled Scallops & Polenta

Please skip this meal if you don't eat scallops.

- 1 pound sea scallops
- ¾ cup polenta cornmeal
- ¾ cup skim milk
- 1 medium Portobello mushroom
- ½ pound green beans
- ¼ cup chopped red onion
- 16 asparagus spear
- 1 teaspoon extra-virgin olive oil

Bring 1½ cups of water and skim milk to rapid boil. Add salt to taste and slowly add polenta while stirring. Reduce heat. Continue stirring until desired consistency is reached. Pour polenta into lightly greased pan. After polenta has cooled cover and refrigerate. Cut chilled polenta into 4 pieces. Grill on medium-hot fire – about two minutes on each side.

Brush Portobello mushroom and asparagus spear with olive oil and place on grill for about 3 minutes on each side.

Grill scallops on medium-hot fire. Turn after two minutes or when first side turns opaque. Grill until second side turns opaque – about another 2 minutes. Don't overcook but test a scallop by cutting to make sure it's cooked through. Salt and pepper to taste.

Serves 4. The food on the plate pictured below totals about 380 Calories.

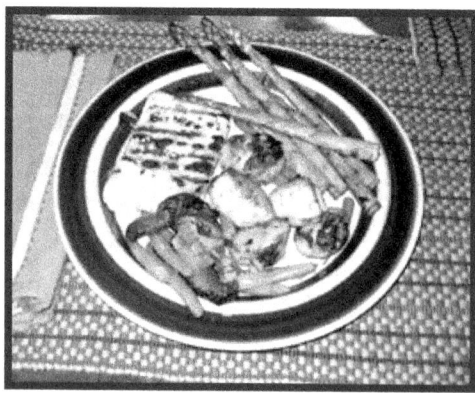

Diet Tip of the Day: To have better control of what you eat **bring your lunch to work**.

Day 65 - Recipe

Frozen Vegetarian Dinner

No recipe today. No cooking today. It's your day off! Some reasonably good frozen vegetarian dinners are:
- Amy's Indian Vegetable Korma (310 Cal)
- Amy's Thai Stir Fry (310 Cal)
- Amy's Asian Noodle Stir Fry (300 Cal)
- Lean Cuisine Veggie Scramble (180 Cal)
- Lean Cuisine Mushroom & Spring Pea Risotto (240 Cal)
- Healthy Choice Asian Potstickers (330 Cal)

Note that if you choose any of the above entrees, you will not use all of the **340 Calories allocated for this meal**. In this case, use the excess 100 or so calories anyway you wish. Splurge on extra dessert or save the calories for another day!

Diet Tip of the Day: **Muscle** is active tissue, fat is not. The more muscle you have, the more calories you burn. Muscle uses a significant number of calories every day for repair and rebuilding, giving your metabolism a boost even when you're resting. So make sure strengthening exercises (like weight lifting) are part of your workout.

Day 66 - Recipe

Pita Pizza

    6 pita bread loaves (Joseph's Flax, Oat Bran & Whole Wheat Pita Bread - 8 oz pkg)
¾ cup part-skim shredded mozzarella, divided
1 large red pepper, sliced
1 medium onion, sliced
6 medium mushrooms, sliced
¾ cup tomato sauce, divided
4 tablespoons olive oil

1) Cook olive oil in large skillet over medium-high heat. Add pepper slices, onion slices and mushroom slices and sauté until they softened.
2) Toast pita loaves slightly (so they don't get soggy when sauce is applied). Coat one side of pita with tomato sauce. Arrange pepper, onion and mushroom slices on individual pita loaves and sprinkle shredded mozzarella cheese on top.
3) In oven preheated to 400°F, place pita loaves on baking tin coated with cooking spray. Cook approximately 5 minutes or until cheese melts. Season with salt and pepper to taste.

Serves 3. 430 Calories per serving (Two Pita Pizzas per serving.)

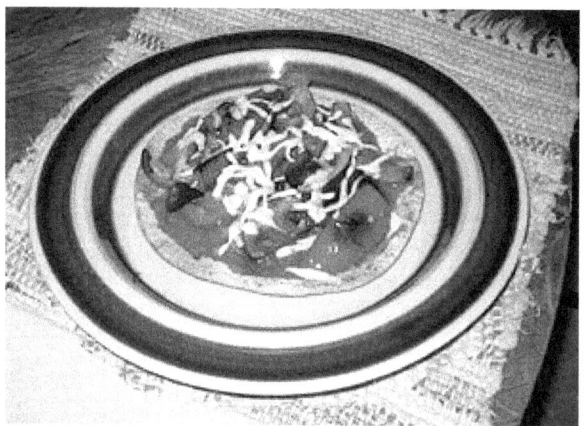

Note only one pita pizza shown. Serving size is <u>two</u> pita pizzas.

Diet Tip of the Day: On a reducing diet, **when you lose – you win**! You win a much better chance for a longer healthier life, you win a sense of well-being, you win a more attractive appearance – and finally you win a feeling of accomplishment.

Day 67 - Recipe

Fish Dinner - Out

No recipe today. No cooking today. Have a fish dinner at your favorite restaurant, but make sure you choose a restaurant where you have a good chance to achieve your calorie goal. For today, your **goal for dinner is a maximum of 595 Calories**. This includes appetizer, soup, main course and dessert.

Tips for Eating Fish Out: The following is almost an exact repeat of the advice given eating out on previous days. First, order simple, such as broiled fish with steamed vegetables and brown rice. Tell the waiter you want no sauce, no gravy, nothing added. Then, knowing your calorie objective, and that fish is about 50 Calories per ounce, most steamed vegetable servings average approximately 50 Calories per cup, and rice is about 100 Calories per ½ cup, decide how much to eat – and take the remainder home. If fresh fruit is not an option, pass on dessert and have the evening snack specified for that day in the diet.

In a restaurant, some nutritionists recommend you eat the low-calorie items on your plate first. Start with the salad, soup and veggies. By the time you get to the fish and starches you will hopefully be full enough to be content with smaller portions of the higher-calorie choices.

Diet Tip of the Day: When you're eating out, consider **ordering children's portions** or a small sandwich as a way to trim calories and get the size of your meals under control.

Day 68 - Recipe

Sorba Noodles & Broccoli Rabe

6 ounces soba noodles or whole grain spaghetti
1 pound broccoli rabe
2 tablespoons extra-virgin olive oil
½ teaspoon sesame seeds
handful fresh cilantro, chopped

Peanut sauce:

½ cup peanut butter
¼ cup reduced sodium soy sauce
3 tablespoons rice vinegar
2 tablespoons honey
1 teaspoon grated fresh ginger
2 cloves garlic, pressed or minced
¼ teaspoon red pepper flakes

1) Prepare broccoli rabe by rinsing well and patting dry. Slice off tough lower stem ends.

2) Prepare peanut sauce: In 2-cup liquid measuring cup, whisk ingredients together with 3 tablespoons water. Set aside.

3) Bring large pot of salted water to boil. Meanwhile, warm 2 tablespoons olive oil in a large skillet over medium heat. Add broccoli rabe and season with a dash of salt and a small pinch of red pepper flakes. Toss to combine and continue cooking, stirring occasionally, until leaves have wilted and stems are easily pierced by a fork, about 8 minutes. Remove from heat.

4) Once water is boiling, add soba noodles and cook until al dente, about 5 minutes. Drain noodles and return them to pot. Add broccoli rabe and toss with peanut sauce.

5) Top individual servings with sprinkle of chopped cilantro & sesame seeds.

Serves 4. About 490 Calories per serving

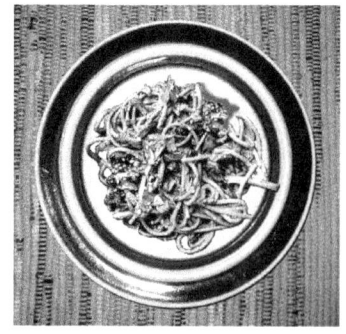

Day 69 - Recipe

Tofu-Veggie Stir Fry

Citrus Sauce:
    6 tablespoons cooking wine
    ¼ cup orange juice
    1 tablespoon light soy sauce
    2 teaspoons toasted sesame oil
    1 teaspoon grated or minced fresh ginger
    1 teaspoon cornstarch
    1 tablespoon toasted sesame seeds

Stir Fry:
    1 (14-ounce) package firm tofu, drained
    1 tablespoon cooking oil
    1½ cups fresh or frozen sugar snap peas
    3 medium carrots, thinly sliced
    ¾ cup thinly sliced onion

1. Stir together sauce ingredients. Set aside while preparing stir fry.
2. Press and pat tofu dry with a towel to remove excess water. Cut into ½-inch cubes.
3. Heat a large skillet or wok over medium-high heat. Add oil and tofu; stir frequently until tofu is lightly browned, about 5 minutes. Add snow peas, carrots and onion. Stir-fry about 5 minutes until vegetables are cooked, but still crisp.
4. Stir in prepared sauce and cook 1-2 minutes until sauce is slightly thickened. Serve immediately.

Serves 4. 230 Calories per serving

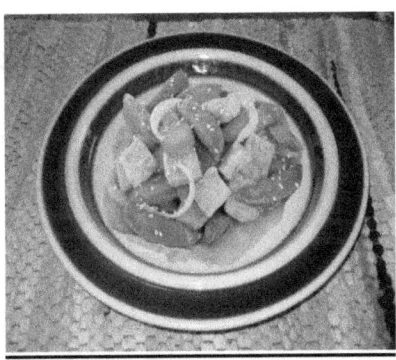

Diet Tip of the Day: Many nutritionists recommend that you buy local and **organic** (if you can afford it).

Day 70 - Recipe

Baked Cod

  4 cod fish fillets (4 to 5 ounces each)
  2 tablespoons flour
  2 tablespoons cornmeal
  2 tablespoons minced fresh herbs
  2 teaspoons lemon juice

Sprinkle cod with lemon juice. Mix flour, cornmeal and herbs and dust the cod with the cornmeal-herb mixture. Bake in oven at 375 °F for 10 minutes. Add salt and black pepper to taste.

Serves 4. One serving is 230 Calories (cod only).

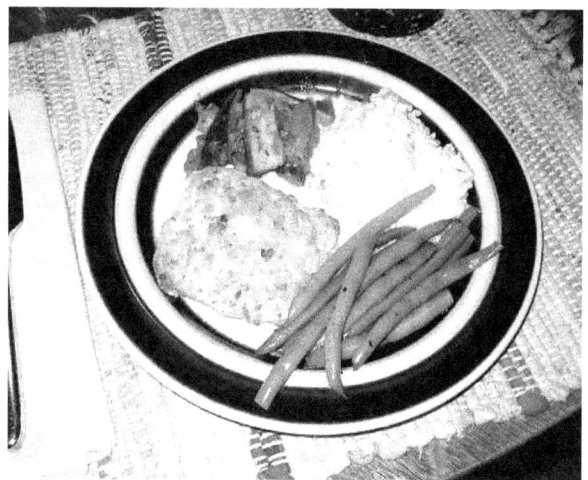

Diet Tip of the Day: It's worth **buying organic** for the "dirty dozen": peaches, strawberries, nectarines, apples, spinach, celery, pears, sweet bell peppers, cherries, potatoes, lettuce, and imported grapes. These fragile fruits and vegetables often require more pesticides to fight off bugs.

Day 71 - Recipe

Tortellini Pasta & Beans

1 9-ounce refrigerated package cheese-filled spinach tortellini
1 15-ounce can cannellini (white kidney) beans, rinsed and drained
¾ cup crumbled garlic-and-herb-flavored feta cheese (3 ounces)
2 tablespoons olive oil
1 large tomato, chopped
4 cups baby spinach

1) Cook tortellini according to package directions. Drain and return to pan.
2) Add drained beans, feta cheese, and olive oil to tortellini in saucepan. Cook over medium heat until beans are hot and cheese begins to melt, gently stirring occasionally. Add tomato; cook another minute. Sprinkle black pepper.
3) Divide spinach among four dinner plates. Top with tortellini mixture.

Serves 4. 450 Calories per serving

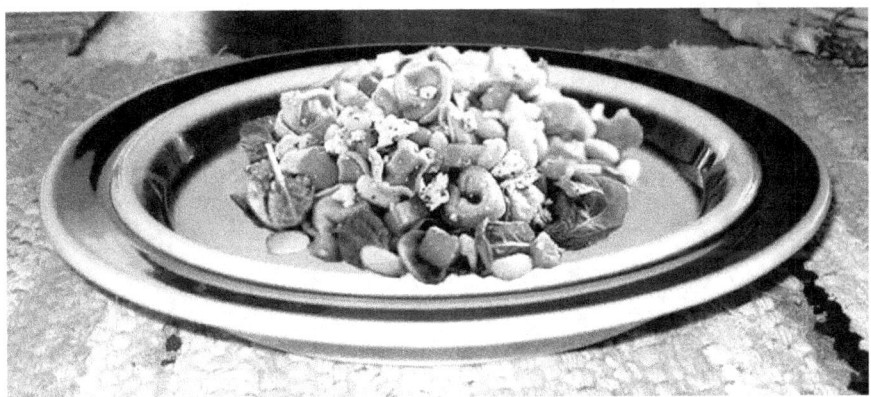

Diet Tip of the Day: Nutritionists define a "**junk food**" as a food that offers little if any essential nutrients – except calories – and when eaten it replaces more important foods.

Day 72 - Recipe

Pasta-Based Dinner - Out

No recipe today. No cooking today. Have a pasta dinner at your favorite Italian restaurant, but make sure you choose a restaurant where you have a reasonable chance to achieve your calorie goal. For today, **your goal for dinner is a maximum of 640 Calories**. This includes any appetizer, soup, main course and any dessert.

Tips for Eating Pasta: Americans adore Italian food. But you can consume a lot of calories in an Italian restaurant – if you order carelessly. For example a typical portion of Fried calamari with garlic bread totals more than 1,100 Calories!

First rule, order simple. Look for pasta in a marinara sauce and a salad with dressing on the side. Then, knowing your 640 Calorie objective, and that most pastas are about 50 Calories per ounce, and marinara tomato sauce averages about 70 Calories per half cup, decide how much of the meal you can eat – and take the remainder home. To stay within your maximum allowable calorie total, you should pass on dessert and have the evening snack specified for that day in the diet.

Diet Tip of the Day: In the U.S., we consume more than 100 pounds of **sugar** per year per person, totaling an unhealthy, nutritionally empty, 500 Calories per day. This large intake of sugar leads to obvious ills, such as obesity and tooth decay.

Day 73 - Recipe

<u>Frozen-Fish Dinner</u>

No recipe today. No cooking today. It's your day off! Some reasonably good frozen fish dinners are:
- Lean Cuisine Shrimp Alfredo (200 Cal)
- Lean Cuisine Parmesan Crusted Fish (290 Cal)
- Lean Cuisine Salmon with Basil (250 Cal)
- Healthy Choice Herb-Crusted Fish (270 Cal)

That's it. At this writing, there are just not that many frozen fish dinners for sale at supermarkets, although new entrees are being introduced continually. If you choose any of the above entrees, you will not use all of the **300 Calories allocated for this meal**. In this case, use the excess 100 or so calories anyway you wish. Splurge on extra dessert or save the calories for another day!

Please read the important **Frozen-Food Safety Warning** in **Appendix C** on page 209.

<u>**Diet Tip of the Day:**</u> Thinking about using **honey** rather than sugar? Honey has about 21 calories per teaspoon while sugar has 15. And the vitamin and mineral content of honey is very low.

Day 74 - Recipe

Pasta Pomodoro

Pasta Pomodoro (Italian for pasta with tomatoes) is typically prepared with angel hair pasta, olive oil, fresh tomatoes, and fresh basil. It's light, delicious and easy to make.

- ¾   pound angel hair pasta
- 1½ pints cherry tomatoes (about 45), halved
- 8   fresh basil leaves, chopped
- 4   cloves garlic, minced
- 2   tablespoons olive oil
- 4   Tbsp grated parmesan cheese

Cook angel hair pasta per package directions. Over medium heat, sauté the garlic in olive oil until it just starts to turn golden. Add tomatoes and cook for about 10 minutes, or until they just start to release juices. Turn off the heat and stir basil into the sauce. Over the cooked pasta, spoon the tomato sauce with a little of the pasta water and garnish with more basil and grated cheese.

Serves 4. 420 Calories per serving

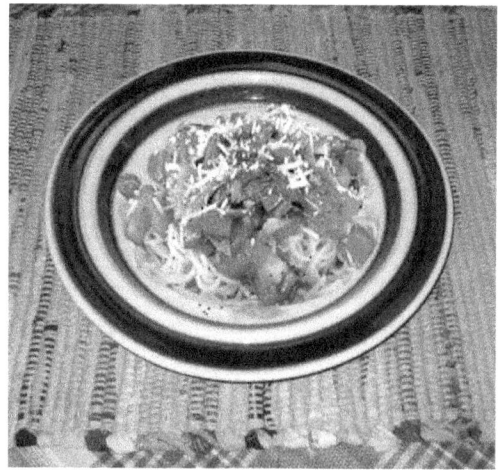

Above prepared with mix of cherry and plum tomatoes.

Diet Tip of the Day: Many health care professionals think that eating a healthy **vegetarian diet** is one of the best things you can do for your short-term and long-term health. But a vegetarian diet must be carefully planned.

Day 75 - Recipe

Spaghetti Squash & Cheese

1½-pound spaghetti squash
2 cups grape tomatoes
4 teaspoons olive oil
2 teaspoons minced garlic
4 teaspoons whole-wheat bread crumbs
1¾ cups 2% milk
½ teaspoon kosher salt
½ teaspoon freshly ground black pepper
3 ounces part-skim mozzarella cheese, shredded (about ¾ cup)
1½ ounces Parmesan cheese, grated (about ⅓ cup)
½ cup torn fresh basil leaves

1. Preheat oven to 350°F. Halve the spaghetti squash and deseed. Place both halves in a in a casserole dish (cut-side down) filled with half cup water. Cook about 45 minutes. Allow to cool 10 minutes and then scrape out spaghetti flesh with a fork into a bowl.
2. Preheat broiler to high. Combine tomatoes and 2 teaspoons of oil in a jellyroll pan. Broil 3 minutes or until tomatoes begin to break down.
3. Place a small saucepan over medium heat. Add remaining 2 teaspoons oil to pan; swirl. Add garlic; cook 1 minute, stirring frequently. Stir in flour. Add milk, salt, and black pepper, stirring with a whisk. Bring to a simmer; cook 1 minute or until thickened, stirring frequently. Remove pan from heat; stir in all but 3 tablespoons of the cheeses.
4. Stir cheese mixture into the spaghetti squash then place in a small 2 quart baking dish. Stir in tomato mixture and torn basil. Sprinkle remaining cheeses over spaghetti squash mixture. Broil 2 minutes or until the top is browned. Garnish with basil leaves.

Serves 6. About 300 Calories per serving.

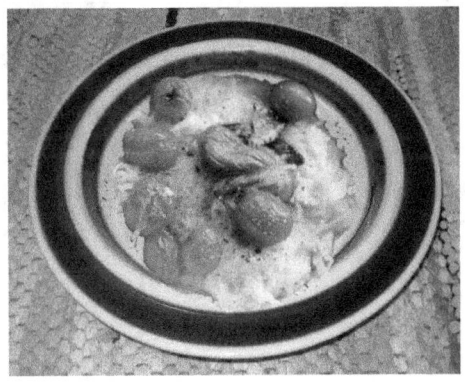

Day 76 - Recipe

Gary & Sue's Grilled Scallops

For Pesceterians that do not eat scallops, please skip this meal.

We were invited to dine with our good friends, Gary and Sue. They prepared a simple, but nutritious low-calorie meal – which featured scallops. (Scallops are a very low calorie food – expensive but great when you're on a diet.) The photo below is our version of the main course they served that night.

- 1½ pounds sea scallops
- 3 medium tomatoes, sliced, divided
- 4 ears of corn
- 2 tablespoons olive oil, divided
- 1 tablespoon balsamic vinegar, divided

Place scallops in a shallow bowl. Add olive oil and vinegar and toss to coat. Grill scallops on medium-hot fire. Turn after two minutes or when first side turns opaque. Grill until second side turns opaque – about another 2 minutes. Don't overcook but test a scallop by cutting to make sure it's cooked through. Salt and black pepper to taste.

Serves 4. The food pictured on the plate below totals about 360 Calories.

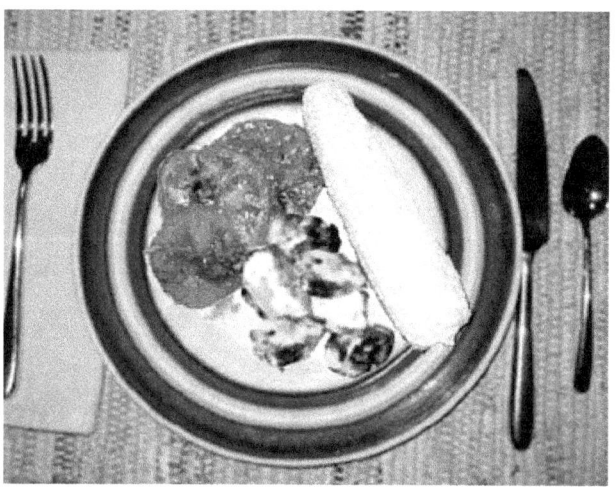

Diet Tip of the Day: When you eat fiber, it simply passes straight through, untouched by but aiding your digestive system. **Zero calories absorbed!**

Day 77 - Recipe

Eggplant Parmesan

3 medium eggplants, cut crosswise into ½-inch slices
3 tablespoons olive oil
1 large onion, finely chopped
1 large clove garlic, thinly sliced
1 ½ teaspoons dried oregano
1 28-ounce can no-salt plum tomatoes or crushed tomatoes
1 tablespoon red wine vinegar
½ cup (packed) fresh basil leaves
½ cup freshly grated Parmesan cheese
⅓ cup fine dry bread crumbs

1. Preheat oven to 450°F. Brush both sides of eggplant slices with olive oil, and place in a single layer on baking sheets. Bake until undersides are golden brown, 10 to 15 minutes, then turn and bake until other sides are lightly browned. Set aside. Reduce oven to 375°F.

2. Meanwhile, in a large saucepan over medium heat, add 2 tablespoons olive oil, onion, oregano and garlic. Sauté until soft, about 10 minutes. Add plum tomatoes and their juices. Break up whole tomatoes. Cover, reduce heat to low and simmer 15 to 20 minutes.

3. Add vinegar, basil and salt and pepper to taste. In a 10-by-6-inch baking pan, spoon a small amount of tomato sauce, then add a thin scattering of parmesan cheese, then a single layer of eggplant. Repeat until all ingredients are used, ending with a little sauce and a sprinkling of parmesan cheese. In a small bowl, combine bread crumbs with enough olive oil to moisten. Sprinkle on top.

4. Bake until eggplant mixture is bubbly and center is hot, 30 to 45 minutes depending on size of pan and thickness of layers. Remove from heat and allow to rest before serving.

Serves 5. About 270 Calories per serving

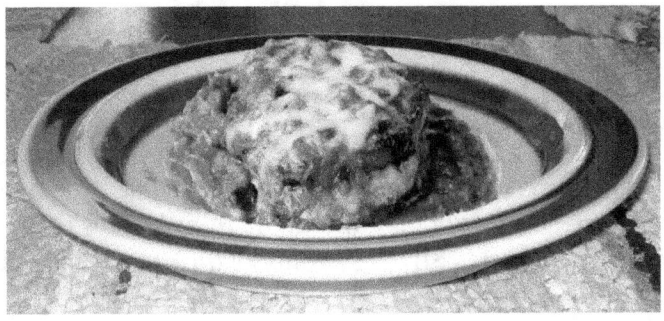

Day 78 - Recipe

Trout with Lemon & Capers

4   trout fillets (4-oz each), skin attached
3   tablespoons unsalted butter, divided
2   tablespoons olive oil
2   tablespoons lemon juice
4   teaspoons chopped parsley
1   teaspoon capers
2   small lemons peeled and segmented

Score 2 crosswise slits (skin deep only) into each trout fillet using sharp knife. Turn the fillets over and season flesh with the salt and pepper.

Heat 1 tablespoon butter and the olive oil in a large nonstick skillet over medium-high heat. Place the fillets in the nonstick skillet, skin side up, and cook until golden brown, about 3 minutes. Turn and continue until cooked through and the skin begins to crisp around edges, about 2 more minutes. Transfer fillets to serving dish and keep warm.

Add the remaining 2 tablespoons butter to the hot skillet and cook until just brown. Stir in the lemon juice, parsley, capers, and lemon segments. Pour sauce over fillets and serve.

Serves 4. 340 Calories per serving (trout and sauce only)

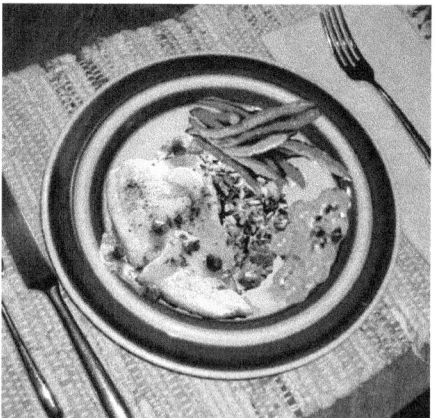

Diet Tip of the Day: Nearly every animal food, including dairy products, eggs, meat, poultry and fish are **complete proteins** because they contain all eight-essential amino acids. Soy is the only plant-based food that has all eight essential-amino acids.

Day 79 - Recipe

Vegetarian Dinner - Out

No recipe today. No cooking today. Have dinner at your favorite vegetarian restaurant, but make sure you choose a restaurant where you have a fighting chance to achieve your calorie goal. For your vegetarian dinner out, your maximum allowable calories (including appetizer, soup, main course and dessert) are as follows:

- For the **1,200 Calorie Diet**: 530 Calories
- For the **1,500 Calorie Diet**: 630 Calories

Tips for Eating Vegetarian Out: First, order simple such as tofu stir fried with vegetables, and brown rice. Tell the waiter you want little to no added sauce or gravy. Estimate the calories in the meal: tofu is about 75 Calories per ounce, most vegetable servings average approximately 50 Calories per cup, rice is about 100 Calories per ½ cup, and add about 150 Calories for the oil used in the stir fry. Then knowing your allowable calorie total for the meal, decide how much to eat – and take the remainder home. If fresh fruit is not an option, pass on dessert and have the evening snack specified for that day on this diet.

In a restaurant, most nutritionists recommend you eat the low-calorie items on your plate first. Start with the salad, soup and veggies. By the time you get to the legumes and starches you will hopefully be full enough to be content with smaller portions of the higher-calorie choices.

Incidentally, if you live in a small town with no vegetarian restaurant, to stay on this diet, have a frozen vegetarian entree. And try to abide by the allowable calorie total.

Finally, some dieticians advise their dieting clients not to eat out. That's right. They believe eating at home is safer. But our thought is you have to eat out eventually so why not learn how while your resolve is high?

Diet Tip of the Day: Know your **daily caloric allowance** whether you are trying to maintain your weight or are on a reducing diet. (See "*Weight Control - U.S. Edition*" a NoPaperPress book where you can determine your daily caloric allowance using unique Weight Maintenance tables.)

Day 80 - Recipe

Vegetable Chili

1 tablespoon olive oil
2 medium carrots, cut into ½-inch pieces
2 medium parsnips, cut into ½-inch pieces
1 medium onion, chopped
2 cans (15-ounces each) red kidney beans, drained
4 teaspoons chili powder
1 can (28-ounce) whole tomatoes in juice
¼ cup fresh cilantro leaves, chopped

In saucepot, heat olive oil on medium-high. Add carrots, parsnips, chopped onion, and cook 6 to 8 minutes or until all vegetables are tender and beginning to brown, stirring occasionally.

Meanwhile, on large plate, mash 1 cup drained beans. Stir chili powder into vegetables in saucepot; cook 1 minute, stirring. Add canned tomatoes with their juice, whole and mashed beans, and 2 cups water. Heat to boiling on high, breaking up tomatoes with spoon. Reduce heat to medium and cook, uncovered for 10 minutes, stirring occasionally. Finally, stir in cilantro and serve.

Serves 4. 360 Calories per serving

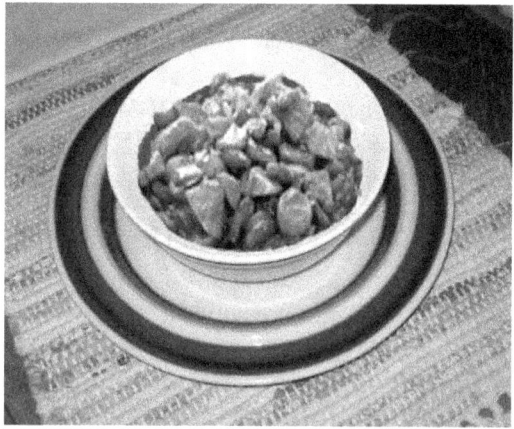

Diet Tip of the Day: **Carbohydrates** provide your body with its basic fuel, the energy your cells need to survive, as well as essential vitamins and minerals, fiber, and other beneficial compounds that promote good health.

Day 81 - Recipe

Frozen Pasta Dinner

No recipe today. No cooking today. It's your day off! Some reasonably good frozen pasta dinners are:

- Lean Cuisine Angel Hair Pomodoro (220 Cal)
- Lean Cuisine Cheese Ravioli (250 Cal)
- Healthy Choice Portobella Spinach Parmesan (230 Cal)
- Healthy Choice Portobella Marsala Pasta (230 Cal)
- Amy's Light & Lean Spagehetti Italiano (240 Cal)

If you choose any of the above entrees, you will not use all of the **300 Calories allocated for this meal**. In this case, use the excess 100 or so calories anyway you wish. Splurge on extra dessert or save the calories for another day!

Please read the important **Frozen-Food Safety Warning** in **Appendix C** on page 209.

Diet Tip of the Day: Keep low-calorie **lean sandwich fixings on hand** (whole-wheat bread, sliced turkey, reduced-fat cheese, lettuce, tomatoes and mustard).

Avocado & Rice Salad

1 cup brown rice
3½ tablespoons dark soy sauce
3½ tablespoons mirin
3½ tablespoons sake
1 tablespoon sugar
1 cup cilantro leaves and tender stems
½ cup peanuts, toasted and roughly chopped
¼ cup pickled ginger, thinly sliced
4 scallions, thinly sliced
2 avocados, peeled, pitted, and thinly sliced
1 cucumber, peeled, seeded, halved lengthwise & sliced into ¼ inch pieces
Zest and juice of 1 lime

1) Rinse rice in strainer under running cold water. Bring 12 cups water to a boil in a large pot with a tight-fitting lid over high heat. Add brown rice, stir once, and boil, uncovered, for 30 minutes. Pour rice into a strainer; cool to room temperature.
2) Teriyaki sauce: Combine soy sauce, mirin, sake, and sugar in a 2-quart saucepan over medium-high heat; cook until sugar has dissolved, 3-5 minutes. Cool sauce slightly.
3) Combine rice, teriyaki sauce, cilantro, peanuts, ginger, scallions, avocados, cucumber, lime zest and juice in a bowl. Plate and garnish with cilantro.
Serves 4. About 410 Calories per serving

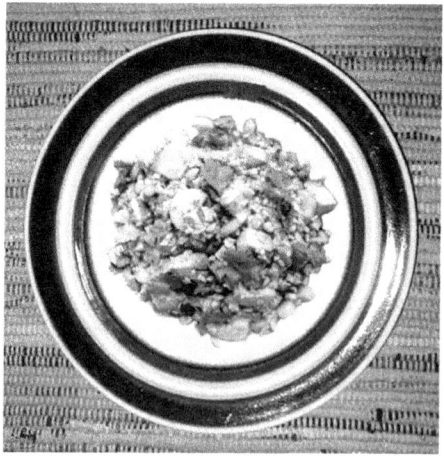

Day 83 - Recipe

Hearty Lentil Stew

½ cup chopped onion
2 garlic cloves, minced
1 tablespoon vegetable oil
1 cup lentils, rinsed
4 tsp vegetable or chicken bouillon granules
3 tsp Worcestershire sauce
1 bay leaf
1 cup chopped carrots
14.5-ounce can diced tomatoes with liquid
10-oz package frozen chopped spinach, thawed
1 Tbsp red wine vinegar

In a large saucepan, sauté onion and garlic in oil until tender. Add 5 cups of water, lentils, bouillon, Worcestershire sauce, ½ teaspoon salt, ¼ teaspoon black pepper and the bay leaf. Bring to a boil. Reduce heat; cover and simmer for 20 minutes.

Add the carrots, tomatoes and spinach; return to a boil. Reduce heat; cover and simmer additional 15 to 20 minutes, or until lentils are tender. Stir in vinegar and serve.

<u>**Serves 4**</u>. 260 Calories per serving

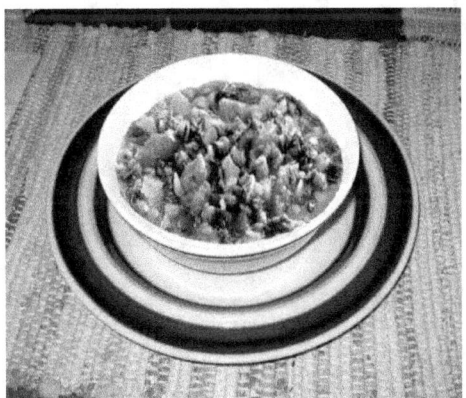

<u>**Diet Tip of the Day:**</u> Monounsaturated fats "**good fats**" are derived from plant sources, such as vegetable oils, nuts, and seeds. This type of fat is found in high concentrations in canola, olive and peanut oils.

Day 84 - Recipe

Black-Eyed Peas over Rice

1 medium onion
2 cups fat-free, lower-sodium vegetable broth
2 cups water
½ teaspoon kosher salt
½ teaspoon freshly ground black pepper
1-pound bag frozen black-eyed peas, thawed
12-ounce bunch fresh turnip greens, trimmed and coarsely chopped
2 tablespoons pepper vinegar

Add chopped onion to a Dutch oven and sauté 4 minutes, stirring occasionally. Stir in broth and the next 6 ingredients (through greens); bring to a boil. Reduce heat, and simmer for about an hour or until peas are tender, stirring occasionally and skimming as necessary. Stir in vinegar. Ladle about 1⅓ cups pea mixture into each of 4 bowls.

Serves 4. 280 Calories per serving (does not include rice)

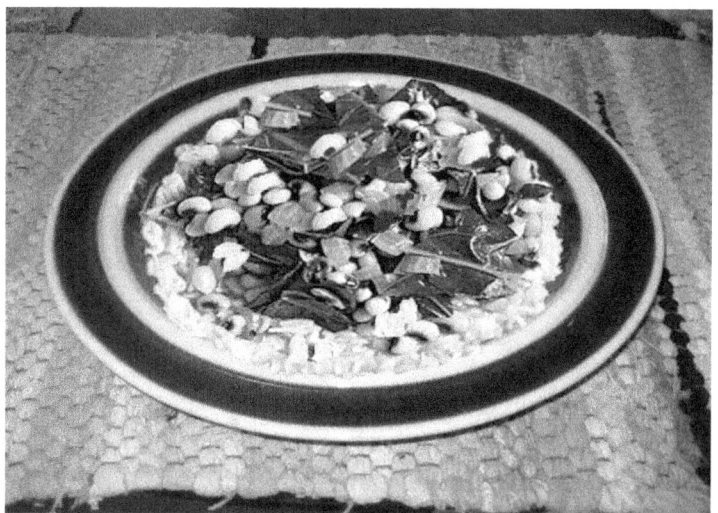

Two servings of black-eyed peas over brown rice on platter.

Diet Tip of the Day: Black-eyed peas are a wonderful food but **black-eyed peas are an incomplete protein**. If however black-eyed peas are eaten with a grain such as rice, the combination forms a complete protein – just as complete a protein as meat, poultry, or fish!

Day 85 - Recipe

<u>Tina's Healthy Frittata</u>

    3 large eggs, plus 3 egg whites
    ¾ cup reduced-fat cottage cheese
    4 ounces smoked gouda cheese, shredded (about 1 cup)
    1 teaspoon minced fresh rosemary
    3 cloves garlic, thinly sliced
    2 tablespoons EVOO
    1 medium onion, chopped
    16-ounce package frozen mixed vegetables, thawed
    2 tablespoons grated parmesan cheese
    1 scant teaspoon paprika

Position a rack in the upper third of your oven and preheat to 450 degrees F. Whisk eggs and egg whites in a bowl. Add the cottage cheese and whisk until almost smooth. Whisk in the gouda and rosemary. In a 10-inch nonstick skillet over medium-high, cook the garlic in the olive oil. Heat until garlic starts to brown, about 1 to 2 minutes. Add onion, season with salt and cook 2 minutes. Add the vegetables, increase the heat to high and cook until just tender, about 5 minutes. Reduce the heat to medium.

Spread the egg mixture evenly in the pan. Cook, without disturbing until a thin crust forms on the bottom, about 2 minutes. Run a rubber spatula around the edge to release egg from the pan. Continue cooking until the bottom is golden, about 2 to 3 minutes. Sprinkle with the parmesan and paprika. Transfer skillet to the oven and bake about 5 to 7 minutes. Remove from the oven, cover and let sit, 5 to 7 minutes. Cut into 4 wedges.
<u>Serves 4</u>. 320 Calories per serving (¼ of frittata)

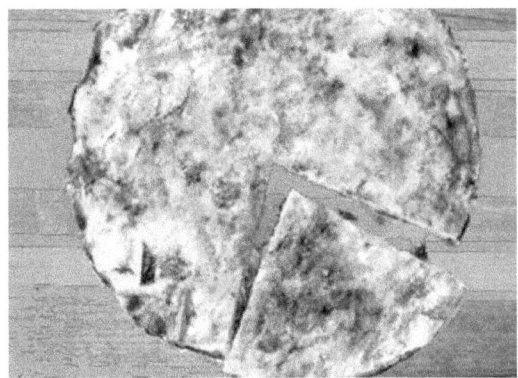

Photo shows frittata on cutting board - hot from skillet.

197

Day 86 - Recipe

Tuna & Bean Salad

1   tuna steak, about 2 inches thick (14 ounces)
2   tablespoons extra-virgin olive oil
1   tablespoon lemon juice
1   garlic clove, crushed
1   tablespoon Dijon mustard
1   15-ounce can cannellini beans, drained
1   small red onion, thinly sliced
2   red peppers, seeded and thinly sliced
½   cucumber, halved lengthwise and thinly sliced
6   cups watercress

Heat a ridged grill pan coated with cooking spray over medium-high heat. Season tuna steak on both sides with coarsely ground black pepper. Cook the tuna 4 minutes on each side - the outside should be browned and the center light pink. Be careful not to overcook. Remove from the pan and set aside.

Mix together the oil, lemon juice, garlic, and mustard in a salad bowl. Season with salt and pepper to taste. Add the cannellini beans, onion, peppers, cucumber and watercress. Toss gently to mix. Cut tuna into ½-inch thick slices. Arrange on top of salad and serve with lemon wedges.

Serves 4. 355 Calories per serving

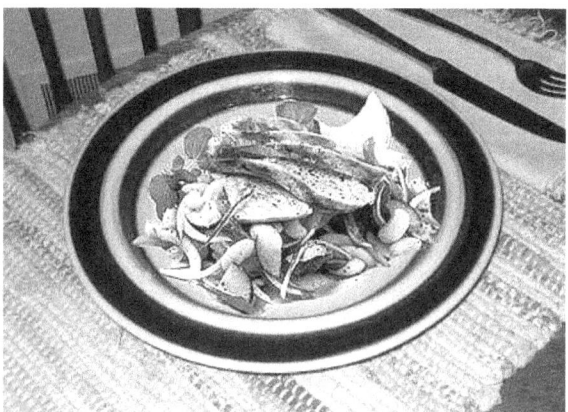

Diet Tip of the Day: In the United States, for a food to be labeled "**whole grain**" it must contain more than 51 percent whole grain by weight.

Day 87 - Recipe

Pasta Primavera

¾ pound penne pasta
2 cups broccoli florets
1 red bell pepper, sliced
1 carrot, cut to 1-inch sticks
½ cup frozen green peas & ½ cup frozen sweet corn
1 small onion, chopped
1 tablespoon minced garlic
3 tablespoons olive oil
1 teaspoon fresh basil, chopped

Cook penne pasta per package directions. Drain and place pasta in a bowl.
Pre-cook the carrot and broccoli florets.

In a large heavy skillet, heat the olive oil and sauté onion and garlic until
lightly golden. Add vegetables and sauté until the peppers are soft.
Combine sautéed vegetables in the bowl with the pasta. Toss well. Garnish
with chopped basil, season to taste, and top with freshly grated Parmesan
cheese.
Serves 4. 460 Calories per serving

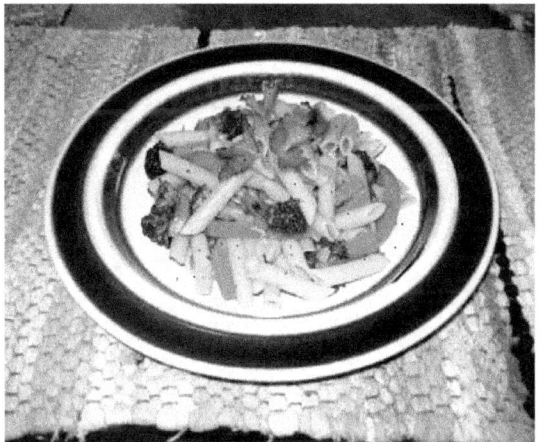

Photo taken before grated cheese was added.

Diet Tip of the Day: When possible, **select fresh and natural foods** and
whole-grain products. Avoid chemical preservatives and additives,
artificial and imitation foods, refined and processed foods, and foods that
are comprised of "nutritionally-empty calories."

Day 88 - Recipe

Frozen Tofu-based Dinner

No recipe today. No cooking today. It's your day off! Some reasonably good frozen tofu-based dinners are:

- Amy's Tofu Scramble (320 Cal)
- Amy's Thai Stir Fry (310 Cal)
- Amy's Teriyaki Bowl (290 Cal)
- Amy's Brown Rice & Vegetables Bowl (260 Cal)

That's it. At this writing, there are just not that many frozen Tofu-based dinners for sale at supermarkets, although there could be new entrees introduced after this book "went to press." If you choose any of the above entrees, you will not use all of the **340 Calories allocated for this meal**. In this case, use the excess 100 or so calories anyway you wish. Splurge on extra dessert or save the calories for another day!

Please read the important **Frozen-Food Safety Warning** in **Appendix C** on page 209.

Diet Tip of the Day: Understand that the only **sure way to slim down for keeps** is to eat less and exercise more. There are no safe short cuts or miracle methods for taking off weight.

Day 89 - Recipe

Fish Stew

For Pesceterians that do not eat shrimp, please skip this meal.

1	pound shrimp, peeled and de-veined
¾	pound skinless flounder fillet, cut into strips
1	pound new baby potatoes, halved
2	peppers (red and yellow) sliced into strips
1	onion, halved and sliced
4	ounces white wine
2	cups vegetable stock
2	cloves garlic, crushed
1	small bunch basil, shredded
1½	tablespoons olive oil

In a large pot, sauté garlic, onion and peppers in olive oil until they are completely softened. Stir in wine, vegetable stock and potatoes. Simmer until potatoes are tender.

Add the shrimp and flounder and cook for additional 4 minutes. Stir in basil and serve.

Serves 4. 300 Calories per serving

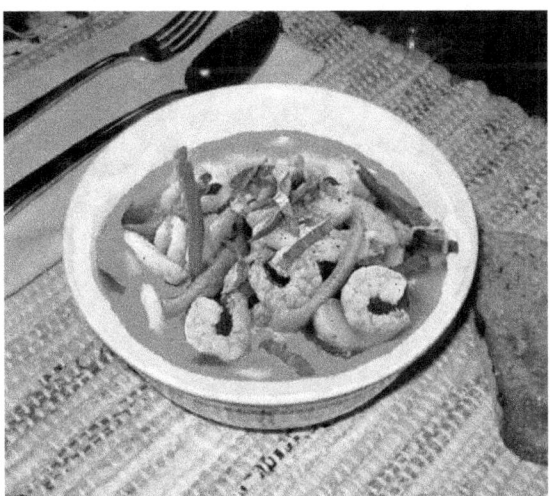

Diet Tip of the Day: All **fish** are relatively low-calorie foods and are good sources of protein and fat-soluble vitamins A and D.

Day 90 - Recipe

Crab Cakes

   1 lb jumbo crab meat
   1½ Tbsp light mayonnaise
   1½ Tbsp chopped green bell pepper
   2   medium green onions, chopped
   1   large egg, beaten
   1   cup panko bread crumbs
   2   Tbsp canola oil
   ¼ tsp black pepper

Drain crab meat on layers of paper towels. Combine crab meat, bell pepper, mayonnaise, black pepper, onions and egg. Stir in ¼ cup panko bread crumbs. (Place remaining panko in shallow dish.)

Divide crab meat mixture into 8 portions. Shape portions into ¾-inch thick patties and dredge in panko. Place non-stick skillet over medium heat and add 1 Tbsp oil. Add dredged patties and cook 3 minutes on each side or until golden.

Prepare remoulade: Combine ¼ cup light mayonnaise, 2 tsp minced shallots, 1 tsp chopped tarragon, 1 tsp chopped parsley, 1½ tsp Dijon mustard and ¾ tsp wine vinegar. Serve remoulade with crab cakes.

Serves 4. 320 Calories per serving (2 crab cakes)

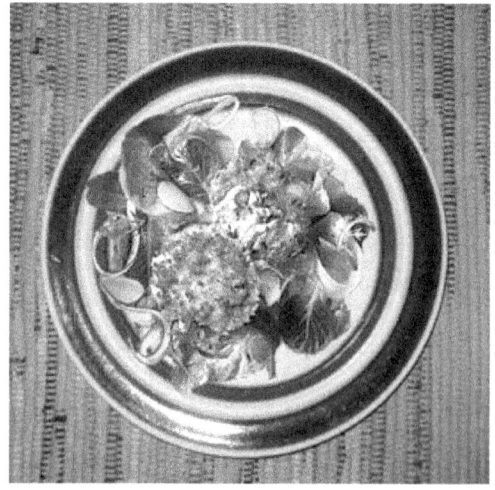

Appendix A
Vegetarian Background
Information

People choose a vegetarian, or plant-based diet, for reasons based on nutrition, health, taste, morality, religion, culture, ethics, aesthetics, environment, economy, or politics.

Vegetarian Benefits

Compared to meat eaters, vegetarians have a lower overall mortality rate and a reduced incidence of heart disease, type 2 diabetes and stroke. And a vegetarian diet has been shown to reduce the risk of some cancers.

Properly planned vegetarian diets have been found to satisfy nutritional needs for all stages of life. Such diets have lower levels of saturated fat and cholesterol and higher levels of carbohydrates, fiber, magnesium, potassium, folate and antioxidants such as vitamins C and E and phytochemicals. And most nutritionists agree that properly planned vegetarian diets are nutritionally adequate and provide health benefits in the prevention and treatment of certain diseases. Large-scale studies have shown vegetarian diets significantly lower the risk of colon cancer, heart disease, high blood pressure and other diseases. In fact, many health-care professionals think that eating a healthy vegetarian diet is one of the best things you can do for your short-term and long-term health. In fact, a well planned vegetarian diet provides the same level of nutrients as a meat-eater's diet.

On the other hand, poorly planned vegetarian diets can increase the risk of cardiovascular disease, blood clots and platelet disorders. (These risks can be offset by sufficient consumption of vitamin B_{12} and polyunsaturated fatty acids.)

Vegetarian Nutrition

Vegetarian, or not, you should always consider the health effects of what you eat. Be sure to replace meat with healthy foods and eat a balanced diet. Eat a variety of whole grains, vegetables and protein foods, such as tofu or veggie burgers to stay full and healthy. While eating an adequate amount of protein is important for vegetarians, getting sufficient calcium and iron (and if you are a vegan vitamin B_{12}) are equally important.

The problem with some vegetarian diets is that they are often relatively low in omega-3 fatty acids and vitamin B_{12}. Conversely, high levels of dietary fiber, folic acid, vitamins C and E, and magnesium, and low consumption of saturated fat are all beneficial aspects of a vegetarian diet.

A well-balanced vegetarian diet with plenty of whole grains, fruits and vegetables is one of the healthiest diets on the planet. You do, however, need to make sure you get ample amounts of the following vital nutrients and micronutrients.

Protein

Most people eat too much protein – not too little of it. Adults need about 0.79 grams of protein for every kilogram of body weight per day to keep from slowly breaking down their own tissue. (That translates as approximately 0.36 grams of protein for every pound of body weight.) A case in point, an adult female weighing 154 pounds (70 kg) requires about (154 x 0.36), or 55 grams of protein per day. An adult male weighing 180 pounds requires (180 x 0.36), or 65 grams per day. How much protein is in food? A few examples: There are approximately seven grams of protein per ounce of beef, poultry, fish, cheese or peanuts. Soybeans pack 10 grams of protein per ounce. Most other beans and lentils contain about six grams of protein per ounce. There are roughly three grams of protein in an ounce of whole-grain cereal, and milk has one gram of protein per fluid ounce.

One cup of tofu contains about 20 grams of protein. Lots of foods contain protein and if vegetarians eat a well-balanced diet, they should undoubtedly consume more than enough protein without even thinking about it. Lacto-ovo vegetarians get sufficient protein from eggs and dairy. Pescaterians get all the protein they need from sea food, eggs and dairy. While vegans can get their protein from tofu, veggie burgers, soy, lentils, chickpeas, nuts and seeds, brown rice and whole grains.

Proteins are composed of amino acids. Often a concern with vegetarian and non-vegetarian is adequate intake of the eight essential amino acids, which cannot be synthesized by humans. While dairy and egg products provide complete protein sources for ovo-lacto vegetarians, several vegetable foods such as, soy, lupin beans, pumpkin seeds, hempseed, chia seeds, amaranth, buckwheat, pistachio nuts, and quinoa, also have significant amounts of all eight types of essential amino acids. Essential amino acids, can also be obtained by eating complementary plant sources that, in combination, provide all eight essential amino acids (e.g. brown rice and beans, whole wheat pasta and beans, or hummus and whole wheat pita,- though combining these in the same meal is not necessary). Protein intake in vegetarian diets is often lower than in meat diets but usually meets the daily requirements of most people. Numerous studies confirm that vegetarian diets supply sufficient protein provided a variety of plant sources are consumed.

Iron

Vegetarian diets typically contain similar levels of iron to non-vegetarian diets, but the iron is often not absorbed as well as iron from meat sources. In addition, iron absorption is sometimes inhibited by other foods in the diet. Some dieticians recommend consuming foods high in vitamin C, such as citrus fruit or juices, tomatoes, or broccoli, as a way to increase the amount of iron absorbed. Vegetarian foods that are rich in iron are black beans, kidney beans, broccoli, lentils, oatmeal, raisins, spinach, cabbage, lettuce, black-eyed peas, soybeans, many breakfast cereals, sunflower seeds, chickpeas, tomato juice, molasses, thyme, and whole-wheat bread. Vegan diets are often higher in iron than lacto-vegetarian diets, because dairy products are low in iron. The American Dietetic Association, asserts that iron deficiency is no more common in vegetarians than in meat eaters, and iron deficiency anemia is rare in all diets.

Vitamin B_{12}

Vitamin B_{12} is not generally found in plants but is occurs naturally in foods of animal origin. Lacto-ovo vegetarians can obtain vitamin B_{12} from dairy products and eggs, while vegans can obtain vitamin B_{12} from a dietary supplement and fortified foods (such as some soy products and breakfast cereals). The recommended dietary allowance for B_{12} in the United States is 2.4 mcg per day and 2.8 mcg per day for lactating females. Although the daily requirement for vitamin B_{12} is very small, a vitamin B_{12} deficiency is very serious and can lead to anemia and irreversible nerve damage.

Fatty Acids

Omega-3 and omega-6 fatty acids are called "essential" fats for good reason. Humans need them for many functions, from building healthy cells to maintaining brain and nerve function. But our bodies cannot produce them. The only source is food. These polyunsaturated fats are also important because they lower the risk of heart disease. Some studies suggest these fats may also protect against type 2 diabetes, Alzheimer's disease, and age-related brain decline. Omega-6 comes from soybean oil, corn oil and sunflower oil, as well as from nuts and seeds. The

American Heart Association recommends that at least 5% to 10% of daily food calories come from omega-6 fatty acids. Omega-3 comes primarily from fatty fish such as salmon, mackerel, and tuna, and in lesser amounts from walnuts and flaxseeds.

Calcium

Calcium intake in vegetarians and vegans can be similar to that in meat eaters, provided the diet is properly planned. Lacto-ovo vegetarians consume dairy products and can obtain calcium from dairy sources like milk, yogurt, and cheese. Non-dairy milks that are fortified with calcium, such as soymilk and almond milk also contribute a significant amount of calcium to the diet. The calcium found in broccoli, bok choy, and kale is also well absorbed by the body. Though the calcium content per serving is lower in these vegetables than in a glass of milk, the absorption of the calcium is higher. Other foods that contain calcium include calcium-set tofu, blackstrap molasses, turnip greens, mustard greens, soybeans, almonds, okra, and dried figs. Although calcium is found in spinach, Swiss chard, beans and beet greens, the calcium in these foods is poorly absorbed by humans.

Vitamin D

Vitamin D is found in many foods, including fish, eggs, fortified milk, and cod liver oil. In addition, 10 minutes of sensible daily sun exposure is sufficient to prevent vitamin D deficiency. Vitamin D comes in several different types. Two forms are important to humans: vitamin D2, which is made by plants, and vitamin D3, which is made by human skin when exposed to sunlight. Foods may also be fortified with vitamin D2 or D3. The major role of vitamin D is to maintain normal blood levels of calcium and phosphorus. Vitamin D helps the body absorb calcium, which forms and maintains strong bones. It is used alone or together with calcium to improve bone health and decrease fractures. Vitamin D is thought to also protect against osteoporosis, high blood pressure, cancer, and other diseases.

Tofu Info

Tofu is an excellent non-animal high-protein food made from soybeans that is frequently linked with vegetarianism. Tofu comes in two basic varieties: soft or silken tofu and firm or regular tofu. Tofu has no taste but readily absorbs the flavor of other foods. Refrigerate tofu after you open a package and use it within four days.

Firm versions of tofu (well-drained) are used for kebabs, mock meats, and dishes requiring a consistency that holds together, while the softer tofu styles are used in desserts, soups, shakes, and sauces. Grated firm western tofu is sometimes used as a meat substitute and can be barbecued because it will hold together on a barbecue grill. Soft tofu is sometimes used as a dairy-free or low-calorie filler. Silken tofu may be used to replace cheese in certain dishes such as lasagna.

Most proteins are delicious even when seasoned simply with salt and pepper. Not tofu which most often tofu tastes bland. But you can turn it into a food you actually want to eat with the following tips.

Buying Tofu
Tofu is usually found in a refrigerated case in the produce department (fruit and vegetables) of most supermarkets. Some stores have tofu in the dairy section and others in stock it in health-food.

Preparing Tofu
1) Most tofu comes packed in water. But a water-logged block of tofu won't absorb a marinade or get crispy in a frying pan. The first thing to do is drain the block as much as possible. To drain it, slice the block and place the slices on a paper towel-lined baking sheet. Top tofu with more paper towels and then a heavy object. Let tofu sit at least one hour. Once drained, you can marinate the tofu or start cooking it.
2) After pressing, tofu is ready to absorb flavor. But the tofu still retains some water and oil and water don't mix. In most cases, use soy, citrus, or vinegar-based marinades instead.
3) Trying to get tofu crispy is difficult. Tossing tofu in cornstarch overcomes the difficulty. Place cornstarch in a bowl, add drained or marinated tofu pieces, and toss. A light coating is best.
4) To sear tofu, use sesame oil which can take the heat and doubles as a flavoring agent, giving the tofu a nutty flavor.

Leftover Tofu
Once a package of tofu is opened it will last about three days if refrigerated. You can freeze leftover tofu. Frozen tofu can last up to three months. And you can freeze any kind of tofu: silken, firm, or extra-firm. Just cut the tofu into cubes and freeze the cubes on a baking sheet. Once hard, store the tofu together in a freezer container. Thaw leftover tofu on a counter top during dinner prep. Thawed tofu can be cooked just as fresh tofu. But squeeze the tofu gently before cooking to eliminate extra moisture.

Appendix B
Vegetarian Soup*

The following lists soup selections that come in cans and microwavable bowls. See the important note at the end of list regarding serving size. Valid as of 07/30/20.

Soup Description	Container	Calories
Amy's Organic Chunky Vegetable	Canned	60
Healthy Choice Cheese Tortellini	Microwaveable	90
Amy's Organic Minestrone	Canned	90
Amy's Organic Split Pea	Canned	100
Amy's No Chicken Noodle	Canned	100
Amy's Organic Butternut Squash	Canned	100
Healthy Choice Country Vegetable	Microwaveable	100
Amy's Organic Vegan Chunky Tomato	Canned	110
Healthy Choice Red Bean and Rice	Microwaveable	130
Healthy Choice Tomato Basil	Microwaveable	130
Amy's Organic Hearty Spanish Rice &	Canned	140
Amy's Organic Hearty Rustic Italian	Canned	140
Amy's Organic Southwestern	Canned	140
Amy's Organic Thai Coconut	Canned	140
Healthy Choice Vegetable Barley	Microwaveable	140
Amy's Organic Quinoa, Kale & Red	Canned	150
Amy's Organic Lentil Vegetable	Canned	160
Healthy Choice Traditional Lentil	Microwaveable	160
Amy's Indian Golden Lentil	Canned	220

* **Important:** When the Daily Meal Plan menu specifies soup, have only one serving (usually this is 1 cup = 8 ounces) unless stated otherwise.

Appendix C
Frozen Food Safety

Increasingly, food giants like ConAgra, Nestlé and others that supply Americans with processed foods concede that they cannot ensure the safety of their food products. Frozen foods pose a particularly serious safety problem because unsuspecting consumers buy frozen foods for their convenience and incorrectly believe that cooking frozen foods is a matter of taste – not safety.

Still the food industry says that extensive outbreaks of food-borne illness are rare, even though it is well-known that most of the millions of cases of food-borne illness every year go unreported or are not traced to the source. For example, each year approximately 40,000 cases of salmonella poisoning are reported in the United States – but perhaps as many as one million cases go unreported. (Salmonella is a type of bacteria most often found in poultry, eggs, unprocessed milk, meat and water.) Recently salmonella pathogens in some frozen meals have sickened thousands of people.

How could this happen? First, the supply chain for ingredients in processed foods – from flour to fruits and vegetables to flavorings – is becoming more complex and global in the drive to keep food costs down. As a result, government and industry officials concede that almost every food ingredient is now a potential carrier of pathogens. A further complication is that a large number of food companies subcontract processing work to save money and don't require suppliers to test for pathogens. In fact, companies often don't even know who is supplying their ingredients.

In addition, many frozen-food manufacturers have stopped cooking their products at high temperatures, a tactic they call the "kill step," which is intended to eliminate any lingering microbes. Frequently this process step turns some of the frozen food ingredients into mush. So, instead the "kill step" has been shifted to consumers. For example, ConAgra has added food safety instructions to its frozen meals, including the Healthy Choice brand. A typical "frozen-food safety" instruction offers this guidance: "Internal temperature needs to reach 165°F as measured by a food thermometer in several spots."

Moreover, General Mills, now advises consumers to avoid microwaves altogether and cook their frozen pizzas only in a conventional oven.

Bottom line: To be safe, always cook frozen foods so that the internal temperature reaches 165°F as measured by a good food thermometer.

NoPaperPress eBooks and Paperbacks

100-Day Super Diet-1200 Cal*
100-Day Super Diet-1500 Cal*
100-Day No-Cooking Diet-1200 Cal*
100-Day No-Cooking Diet-1500 Cal*
90-Day Smart Diet-1200 Cal*
90-Day Smart Diet-1500 Cal*
90-Day No-Cooking Diet - 1200 Cal*
90-Day No-Cooking Diet - 1500 Cal*
90-Day Perfect Diet - 1200 Cal*
90-Day Perfect Diet - 1500 Cal*
60-Day Perfect Diet-1200 Cal*
60-Day Perfect Diet-1500 Cal*
50-Day Flex Diet-1200 Cal*
50-Day Flex Diet-1500 Cal*
30-Day Quick Diet - Women*
30-Day Quick Diet for Men*
30-Day No-Cooking Diet*
30-Day Diet - Women - Metric*
30-Day Diet for Men - Metric*
25 Day Easy Diet-1200 Cal*
25 Day Easy Diet-1500 Cal*
25-Day No-Cooking Diet
10-Day Express Diet
10-Day No-Cooking Diet*
7-Day Diet for Women*
7-Day Diet for Men*
7-Day No-Cooking Diets*
90-Day Gluten-Free Diet-1200 Cal*
90-Day Gluten-Free Diet-1500 Cal*
30-Day Gluten-Free Quick Diet*
30-Day Gluten-Free No-Cooking Diet*
7-Day Diet for Women - Metric*
7-Day Diet for Men - Metric
7-Day Gluten-Free Express Diet*
7-Day Gluten-Free No-Cooking Diet*
90-Day Vegetarian Diet-1200 Cal*
90-Day Vegetarian Diet-1500 Cal*
30-Day Vegetarian Diet*
7-Day Vegetarian Diet*
Weight Loss for Women*
Weight Loss for Women - Metric
Weight Loss for Women - UK
Weight Loss for Men*
Maximum Weight Loss - 1200 Cal*
Maximum Weight Loss - 1500 Cal*

Weight Loss for Men - Metric*
Maximum Weight Loss- 1200 Cal*
Maximum Weight Loss- 1500 Cal*
Weight Control - U.S. Edition*
Weight Control - Metric. Edition
Prof Weight Control Women - U.S.
Prof Weight Control Women - Metric
Prof Weight Control Men - U.S.
Prof Weight Control Men - Metric
Weight Maintenance - U.S. Ed*
Weight Maintenance - Metric. Ed*
Weight Maintenance - UK Ed
Weight Loss for Senior Men*
Weight Loss for Senior Women*
Eat Smart - U.S. Edition*
Eat Smart - Metric Edition
30-Day Mediterranean Diet
Exercise Smart - U.S. Edition*
Exercise Smart - Metric Edition
Exercise Smart - UK Edition*
Total Fitness - U.S. Edition
Total Fitness - Metric Edition
Total Fitness - UK Edition
Total Fitness for Women-U.S. Ed*
Total Fitness for Women - Metric
Total Fitness for Women - UK Ed
Total Fitness for Men - U.S. Ed*
Total Fitness for Men- Metric Ed*
Total Fitness for Men - UK Ed
Senior Fitness - U.S. Edition*
Senior Fitness - Metric Edition*
Senior Fitness - UK Edition*
Computer Diet - U.S. Edition*
Computer Diet - Metric Ed*
Reliable Weight Loss - U.S. Ed
101 Weight Loss Tips*
101 Healthy Eating Tips*
101 Lifelong Fitness Tips*
101 Weight Maintenance Tips
101 Weight Loss Recipes
101 GF Weight Loss Recipes
101 Veggie Weight Loss Recipes*
30-Day Mediterranean Diet*
90-Day Mediterranean Diet - 1200 Cal*
90-Day Mediterranean Diet - 1500 Cal*

* These titles are available as both ebooks and paperbacks. Our ebooks are sold by Amazon, Apple, Google, Barnes & Noble and Kobo, but our paperbacks are only sold by Amazon.

Disclaimer

This book offers general meal planning, nutrition and weight control information. It is not a medical manual and the author does not claim to be medically qualified. The material in this book is not intended to be a substitute for medical counseling. Everyone should have a medical checkup before beginning a weight loss program. Moreover, the physician conducting the medical exam should be made aware of and should approve the specific weight control program planned. Additionally, while the author and publisher have made every effort to ensure the accuracy of the information in this book, they make no representations or warranties regarding its accuracy or completeness. Where brand-name foods are specified, please check the list of ingredients on the Nutrition Label to assure that the product remains meatless. Further, neither the author nor publisher assume liability for any medical problems that might result from applying the methods in this book, or for any loss of profit, or any other commercial damages, including but not limited to special, incidental, consequential or other damages, and any such liability is hereby expressly disclaimed.